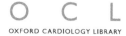

O C L
OXFORD CARDIOLOGY LIBRARY

Hypertension

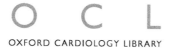

OXFORD CARDIOLOGY LIBRARY

Hypertension

Second Edition

Edited by

Sunil Nadar

Senior Consultant Cardiologist, Sultan Qaboos University Hospital, Muscat, Oman

Gregory YH Lip

Professor of Cardiovascular Medicine, University of Birmingham, UK; and Adjunct Professor of Cardiovascular Sciences, Thrombosis Research Unit, Aalborg University, Denmark

Visiting Professor of Haemostasis Thrombosis & Vascular Sciences, Aston University, Birmingham, UK; Visiting Professor of Cardiology, University of Belgrade, Serbia

OXFORD
UNIVERSITY PRESS

OXFORD
UNIVERSITY PRESS

Great Clarendon Street, Oxford, OX2 6DP,
United Kingdom

Oxford University Press is a department of the University of Oxford.
It furthers the University's objective of excellence in research, scholarship,
and education by publishing worldwide. Oxford is a registered trade mark of
Oxford University Press in the UK and in certain other countries

First Edition published in 2009
Second Edition published in 2015

Impression: 1

Published in the United States of America by Oxford University Press
198 Madison Avenue, New York, NY 10016, United States of America

British Library Cataloguing in Publication Data

Data available

Library of Congress Control Number: 2015938191

ISBN 978–0–19–870197–2

Printed and bound in Great Britain by
Ashford Colour Press Ltd, Gosport, Hampshire

Acknowledgement to first edition contributors

The editors would like to thank the first edition authors whose excellent text and contributions have been continued into this second edition:

Deepak Goyal
Timothy Watson
Ayush Khurana
Jaspal Taggar
Girish Dwivedi
Shridhar Dwivedi
John Kurien

Contents

Contributors

Mehmood Sadiq Butt, Consultant interventional cardiologist, University Hospital Wales, Cardiff, UK

Pravin Jha, South West Yorkshire Partnership NHS Foundation Trust, Mount Vernon Hospital, Barnsley S70 4DP

VJ Karthikeyan, Consultant, Interventional Cardiology, North Wales Cardiac Centre, Glan Clwyd Hospital, Rhyl, UK

Mohammad Khan, Speciality Doctor, South West Yorkshire Partnership NHS Foundation Trust, Mount Vernon Hospital, Barnsley S70 4DP

Gregory YH Lip, Professor of Cardiovascular Medicine, University of Birmingham, UK; Adjunct Professor of Cardiovascular Sciences, Thrombosis Research Unit, Aalborg University, Denmark; Visiting Professor of Haemostasis Thrombosis & Vascular Sciences, Aston University, Birmingham, UK; Visiting Professor of Cardiology, University of Belgrade, Serbia

Sunil Nadar, Senior Consultant Cardiologist, Sultan Qaboos University Hospital, Muscat, Oman

Rajesh Nambiar, Consultant cardiologist, Amarillo Heart Group, Amarillo, Texas, USA

Shankar BG Patil, Department of Cardiology, Leeds Teaching Hospital, Leeds, UK

Vasudevan A Raghavan, Chief Executive Officer, Cardio-metabolic Clinic & Research center; Medical Director, Heart & Hormonal Health Clinic, Round Rock, TX 78681

Kully Sandhu, Cardiology Specialist Registrar, Royal Stoke Hospital, University Hospitals of North Midlands NHS Trust

Muzahir H Tayebjee, Consultant Cardiologist, Leeds Teaching Hospital, Leeds, UK

Viji Samuel Thomson, Department of Cardiology, Christian Medical College and Hospital, Vellore, India

Shamil Yusuf, Consultant Cardiologist and Cardiac Electrophysiologist, Heart of England (NHS) Foundation Trust, Birmingham, UK

List of symbols and abbreviations

ABCD	Appropriate Blood Pressure Control in Diabetes
ACE	angiotensin-converting enzyme
ACEI	angiotensin-converting enzyme inhibitors
ACTH	adrenocorticotrophic hormone
ADA	American Diabetes Association
ADH	anti-diuretic hormone
AFP	alpha feto protein
Aldo	Aldosterone
ALLHAT	Antihypertensive and Lipid Lowering Treatment to Prevent Heart Attack Trial
ANBP-2	Australian National Blood Pressure Study
ANP	atrial natriuretic peptides
ARBs	angiotensin receptor blockers
ARR	absolute risk reduction
AV	Arteriovenous
AVP	argenine vasopressin
BHS	British Hypertension Society
BMI	body mass index
BNP	brain natriuretic peptides
BP	blood pressure
CAD	coronary artery disease
CAFE	conduit artery functional endpoint
CAPP	Captopril Prevention Project
CCBs	calcium-channel blockers
CHARM	Candesartan in Heart Reduction in Mortality and Morbidity
CI	confidence interval
CIBIS-II	Cardiac Insufficiency Bisoprolol Study II
CNP	C-type natriuretic peptides
COER	controlled-onset extended-release
CONVINCE	Controlled ONset Verapamil INvestigation of Cardiovascular Endpoints
CPAP	continuous positive airways pressure
CT	computed tomography
DASH	dietary approaches to stop hypertension
DCT	distal convoluted tubule
DETAIL	Diabetics Exposed to Telmisartan And enalaprIL

DIC	disseminated intravascular coagulation
DM	diabetes mellitus
DSA	digital subtraction angiogram
ECG	Electrocardiography
ELITE	Evaluation of Losartan In The Elderly
ENaC	epithelial sodium channel
ESC	European Society of Cardiology
ESH	European Society of Hypertension
ESRD	end-stage renal disease
EUROPA	European trial On Reduction of Cardiac Events with Perindopril in Stable Coronary Artery Disease
GEMINI	Glycemic Effects in diabetes Mellitus Carvedilol-Metoprolol comparison in hypertensives
GRA	glucocorticoid remediable hyperaldosteronism
GUSTO	Global Utilisation of Streptokinase and Tissue plasminogen activator for Occluded coronary arteries
HCG	human chorionic gonadotrophin
HOPE	Heart Outcomes Prevention Evaluation
HOT	Hypertension Optimal Treatment
HR	hazard ratio
HTn	hypertension
HYVET	Hypertension in the very elderly trial
IDDM	insulin dependent diabetes mellitus
IDNT	Irbesartan Diabetic Nephropathy Trial
IR	insulin resistance
INSIGHT	International Nifedipine GITS Study of Intervention as a Goal in Hypertension Treatment
INTERMAP	International Study of Macro- and Micro-nutrients and Blood Pressure
INTERSALT	The International study of Salt and Blood pressure
INVEST	International Verapamil Trandolapril Study
ISA	intrinsic sympathomimetic activity
ISH	International Society of Hypertension
ISIS	International study of Infarct Survival
IVSd	interventricular septal thickness in diastole
JGA	juxtaglomerular apparatus
JNC	Joint National Committee
JNC-7	Seventh Joint National Committee
LIFE	Losartan Intervention for Endpoint reduction in Hypertension
LIVE	LVH regression Indapamide Enalapril
LV	left ventricular
LVH	left ventricular hypertrophy

LVIDd	left ventricular internal diameter in diastole
LVMI	LV mass index
LVPDd	left ventricular posterior wall at end diastole
MAOIs	monoamine oxidase inhibitors
MARVAL	Microalbuminuria Reduction with VALsartan
MIAMI	Metoprolol In Acute Myocardial Infarction
MERIT-HF	Metoprolol Randomised Intervention Trial in congestive heart failure
MRFIT	multiple risk factor interventional trial
NHBPEP	National High Blood Pressure Education Program
NICE	National Institute for Health and Care Excellence
MAP	Mean Arterial Pressure
MMPs	matrix metalloproteinases
MRA	magnetic resonance angiography
MRC	Medical Research Council
MRI	magnetic resonance imaging
MUFA	monounsaturated fatty acids
NHANES-III	Third National Health and Nutrition Examination Survey
NKF	National Kidney Foundation
NO	nitric oxide
NNt	number needed to treat
NORDIL	NORdic DILtiazem
OPTIMAAL	OPtimal Trial in Myocardial Infarction with the Angiotensin II Antagonist Losartan
tPA	plasminogen activator
PAD	peripheral arterial disease
PAF	
PAI	paroxysmal atrial fibrillation plasminogen activator inhibitor
PATHS	Prevention And Treatment of Hypertension Study
PEACE	Prevention of Events with Angiotensin-Converting Enzyme Inhibition
PHA	Primary hyperaldosteronism
PRA	plasma renin activity
PRESERVE	Prospective Randomized Enalapril Study Evaluating Regression of Ventricular Enlargement
PROGRESS	Perindopril Protection Against Recurrent Stroke Study
PCT	Proximal Convoluted Tubule
PTCA	Percutaneous transluminal coronary angioplasty
PUFA	polyunsaturated fatty acids
QUIET	Quinapril Ischemic Event Trial
RAS	renal artery stenosis
RAAS	Renin–Angiotensin–Aldosterone System

RENAAL	Reduction of Endpoints in NIDDM with the Angiotensin II Antagonist Losartan
RVHT	Renovascular hypertension
RWT	relative wall thickness
SCAT	Simvastatin/Enalapril Coronary Atherosclerosis
SCOPE	Study on Cognition and Prognosis in the Elderly
SGA	small-for-gestational-age
SHEP	Systolic Hypertension in the Elderly Program
SOLVD	Studies Of Left Ventricular Dysfunction
STOP	Swedish Trial in Old Patients
Syst-China	Systolic hypertension study in China
Syst-Eur	Systolic hypertension in Europe Study
TAL	thick ascending LIMB
TARGET	Telmisartan Alone and in Combination with Ramipril Global Endpoint Trial
T2DM	type 2 diabetes mellitus
TIMI-2B	Thrombolysis In Myocardial Infraction
TIMPs	Tissue inhibitors of MMPs
TOD	target organ damage
TONE	Trial of Non-pharmacologic Interventions in the Elderly
tPA	tissue plasminogen activator
TRACE	TRAndolapril Cardiac Evaluation
VALUE	Valsartan Antihypertensive Long-term Use Evaluation Trial
Val-Heft	Valsartan Heart Failure Trial
VALIANT	VALsartan In Acute Myocardial INfarction Trial
VEGF	vascular endothelial growth factor
VMA	vanillymandelic acid
WHO	World Health Organisation
ZGHP	zona glomerulosa hyperplasia

Part 1

Epidemiology, pathogenesis, and diagnosis

Chapter 1

Epidemiology of hypertension

Sunil Nadar

Key points

- Hypertension is a very common condition with a high risk of future cardiovascular events.
- Many factors influence the prevalence and management of hypertension.
- Lifestyle factors along with genetic influences determine the development of hypertension.
- From a public health point of view, intense screening and patient education are important in the diagnosis, management, and prevention of hypertension.

1.1 Introduction

Hypertension is a global phenomenon and is common to all human populations with the exception of some primitive communities that live in cultural isolation, for example, in the Amazon basin. It accounts for up to 6% of adult deaths worldwide. Some reports suggest that as of 2013, there are 1 billion people worldwide, who might have hypertension. It is believed that there is a global epidemic of yet unknown proportions as abnormally elevated blood pressures are often asymptomatic. Indeed the first diagnosis of hypertension is often made when the individual presents with a myocardial infarction or a stroke. Hypertension is thus rightly often referred to as the 'silent killer'. Yet it was not always thought to be a bad thing. Historically, the term 'benign essential hypertension' reflects the attitudes towards high blood pressure in the early twentieth century.

1.2 Historical perspective

The theories regarding blood circulation and blood pressure go far back in history. In ancient Greece, Hippocrates and Galen knew about arteries and veins. Galen was convinced veins and arteries were not connected and blood flowed both backward and forward from the heart. His teachings were unchallenged for more than 1000 years.

It was only during the Middle Ages that these teachings were challenged and new experiments were conducted and these laid the basis for our modern understanding of the heart and circulation. It was William Harvey in 1616 who first described a one-way circulation of blood and correctly suggested the existence of capillaries. In 1733, Stephen Hales, an English clergyman, was the first person to measure blood pressure, albeit in a horse. Almost 150 years later, Ritter von Basch invented a machine that could measure the blood pressure of a human being in a non-invasive manner. This was the forerunner of the device introduced by Riva-Rocci in 1896, which proved to be a prototype of today's refined instruments. This, along with the invention of the stethoscope by René Laennec, helped Russian scientist NS Korotkoff in 1905 to monitor the pulse whilst the blood pressure cuff was inflated, giving birth to the term 'Korotkoff sounds'.

Before long, patients were having their blood pressure checked, and high blood pressure came to be known as 'hypertension'. At that time it was felt that in certain conditions, this raised blood pressure helped to maintain the perfusion of various organs and was not particularly harmful and hence the term 'benign essential hypertension'; as opposed to 'malignant hypertension', which they thought was very high blood pressures that could result in brain haemorrhage and heart failure.

It was only towards the middle of the twentieth century that various surgical and pharmacological interventions were considered for the treatment of hypertension, although its exact risk was uncertain. Some of the initial surgical procedures that were considered included thoracic sympathectomy and the drug therapy was mainly sedatives. Diuretics were introduced for hypertension in the 1950s and 1960s, but scepticism still persisted in the medical community about the benefit of treating this 'benign essential' condition.

1.3 Hypertension and the cardiovascular risk

It was not until the late 1970s and 1980s that large-scale epidemiological studies, including the Framingham study, clearly demonstrated the association between high blood pressure and cardiovascular risk. At the same time a Veterans Administration study demonstrated that treating hypertensive patients with diuretics appeared to protect them from future events. These studies and especially the more recent prospective studies collaboration (Lewington 2002) have demonstrated that there is an almost linear relationship between blood pressure and cardiovascular and cerebrovascular risk. From the ages 40–69, there is a twofold increase in mortality rates from ischemic heart disease, and more than a twofold increase in stroke mortality for each 20 mmHg of increase in systolic blood pressure and 10 mmHg increase of in diastolic blood pressure. They also found that there is no evidence of a threshold wherein blood pressure is not directly related to risk even at levels as low as 115/75 mmHg. They also conclude that a 10 mmHg higher systolic or 5 mmHg higher diastolic blood pressure would in the long term be associated with about a 30% higher risk of death from ischemic heart disease.

It has also been shown that in people with low blood pressure who are not receiving any antihypertensive therapy, the incidence of cardiovascular disease is less. However, this cannot be used to support the benefits of therapy, as naturally occurring low blood pressure may offer a degree of protection that is not provided by a similarly low blood pressure resulting from antihypertensive therapy. However, many randomized control trials have demonstrated a significant benefit for treating individuals with high blood pressure, especially when they are at a high risk for future cardiovascular events due to co-existing factors.

For an individual patient, the greatest risk is from a higher level of blood pressure. However, for the population at large, the greatest burden from hypertension occurs among people with only minimally elevated blood pressure, as they are more likely to develop overt hypertension in the following years and often the majority of them are picked up once they have had an event. From a public health point of view, it would therefore make more sense to have extensive screening programmes and health education programmes on the importance of healthy lifestyle modifications.

1.4 Prevalence

The exact prevalence of hypertension is not really known, but Kearney and colleagues (2005) estimate a worldwide prevalence of approximately 26% of the adult population with marked differences between countries. Other epidemiologic studies appear to suggest that this prevalence is increasing and a survey in the United States suggests that the prevalence of hypertensives has increased by 15 million to around 65 million over a period of 10 years from 1990 to 2000. A more recent publication by Rogers and colleagues (2012) suggests that there are more than 76 million hypertensives in the USA and more than 1 billion hypertensives worldwide. One of the reasons for this increase is the increasing age of the population and changing lifestyles, including an increase in obesity rates.

Some of the determinants of hypertension include genetic and environmental factors. Epidemiological studies suggest that 20–60% of essential hypertension is inherited. Several genetic polymorphisms which might affect the synthesis of proteins such as angiotensinogen glucocorticoid receptors and kallikrein have been reported. Studies from India show that a positive family history of hypertension and stroke was 1.7 times more common in hypertensive patients than in controls.

Racial differences are seen in the prevalence of hypertension among different ethnic groups within the same community. In the United States, Native American Indians have the same or slightly higher prevalence than the general population whilst the Hispanics have the same or a slightly lower prevalence as the general population. On the other hand, African Americans have among the highest prevalence of hypertension in the world. Genetic differences could play a part here.

Geographical variations have been reported in the prevalence of hypertension within the same ethnic group. For example, in the United Kingdom, prevalence rates were higher in Scotland and Northern England as compared to the rest of the country. Dietary differences and other lifestyle differences such as alcohol consumption, obesity, etc., may account for this difference. Age and sex are the other determinants, with blood pressure increasing with age. Men are also more likely to have higher blood pressure than women during their middle age. Above the age of 60 (after menopause), women and men have similar blood pressure and thereafter (above the age of 70 and 80), women tend to have higher blood pressures.

Figure 1.1 shows a changing trend in the number of hypertensive patients (as a percentage of the population) between the years 1950 and 1990. It is interesting to note that the actual percentage of people between the ages of 45 and 60 with a blood pressure higher than

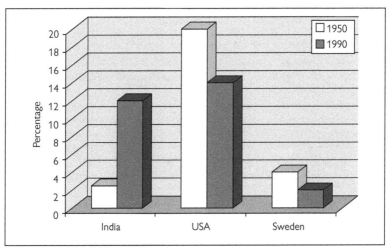

Figure 1.1 Changes in the prevalence of hypertension in adults aged between 45 and 60 in three different countries between 1950 and 1990

140/80 mmHg in the developed world is actually decreasing, whilst it is on the upward trend in India. One of the explanations could be the increasing westernization of the population in India and the adoption of a more sedentary lifestyle coupled with a diet that is richer in fats and salts. This could be in addition to the fact that there is better healthcare now than existed in 1950, and therefore the number of cases that are being diagnosed is increasing.

1.5 **Future prospects**

Our understanding of the pathogenesis of hypertension has improved tremendously over the past few decades. Options for managing hypertension have also increased over this period and they continue to expand at a very fast pace. The current armamentarium of the physician for treating hypertension includes a wide array of drugs such as diuretics, calcium-channel blockers, beta blockers, and antagonists of the renin-angiotensin-aldosterone system. Current dilemmas include whom and when to treat and what drug to initiate treatment with, along with difficulties in knowing what targets to reach.

Our understanding of this interesting subject continues to improve. Until as recently as 1991, scepticism remained about the effectiveness of treating elderly patients with isolated systolic hypertension (> 160/< 90 mmHg). The Systolic Hypertension in the Elderly Program (SHEP) and similar studies have shown decisively that treatment of hypertension (systolic or diastolic) is even more effective in preventing cardiovascular complications in patients aged 60 and older than it is in younger patients.

Some experts have labelled hypertension an 'illness of civilization'. Western culture is associated with stress, poor diet, and lack of exercise and these contribute heavily to the problems of the nearly 50 million Americans who have some form of high blood pressure.

Studies such as the Antihypertensive and Lipid Lowering Treatment to Prevent Heart Attack Trial (ALLHAT) and the Anglo Scandinavian Cardiac Outcomes Trial (ASCOT) have given us a better understanding of the newer antihypertensive agents. Whilst we know that controlling hypertension reduces the risk of cardiovascular events, information from the Third National Health and Nutrition Examination Survey (NHANES-III) highlights the fact that many Americans are not benefiting from this knowledge:

- Only about 70% of people with hypertension in the USA know they have high blood pressure.
- Only about half of people in whom hypertension is diagnosed are being treated with drugs.
- Even when drugs are prescribed, they are frequently misused or abandoned.
- Only 24% of Americans being treated for hypertension maintain systolic blood pressure at 140 mmHg or below and diastolic pressure at less than 90 mmHg.

However, there is room for optimism as well. In the last two decades, mortality from stroke has decreased by almost 60% and deaths from heart attack have been reduced by about half. Fifty years ago, physicians believed stress was a symptom of high blood pressure. Today, many believe the reverse is true, but we have yet to learn the exact mechanisms involved. What actually triggers hypertension in most people? To what extent do genes and the environment contribute to causing hypertension? These are still some of the many unanswered questions in this highly important but often neglected field of medicine.

Key references

Kannel WB (1996). Blood pressure as a cardiovascular risk factor: prevention and treatment. *Journal of American Medical Association*; 275: 1571–76.

Kearney PM, Whelton M, Reynolds K, *et al.* (2005). Global burden of hypertension: analysis of worldwide data. *Lancet;* 365: 217–23.

Lewington S, Clarke R, Qizihash N, *et al.* (2002). Age specific relevance of usual blood pressure to vascular mortality: a meta-analysis of individual data for one million adults in 61 prospective studies. *Lancet;* 360: 1903–13.

National High Blood Pressure Education Programme Working Group report on primary prevention of hypertension (1993). *Archives of Internal Medicine;* 153: 186–208.

Rogers VL, Go AS, Lloyd-Jones DM, *et al.* (2012) On behalf of the American Heart Association Statistics Committee and Stroke Statistics Subcommittee 2012 update: a report from the American Heart Association. *Circulation;* 358: 1682–86

Vasan RS, Larson MG, Leip EP, *et al.* (2001). Assessment of frequency of progression to hypertension in non-hypertensive subjects in the Framingham Heart Study. A cohort study. *Lancet;* 358: 1682–86.

Chapter 2

Pathophysiology of hypertension

Sunil Nadar

Key points

- Hypertension is a complex disease with many factors contributing to its development and maintenance.
- Increased circulatory volume and increased peripheral resistance are the main pathophysiological mechanisms.
- The renin–angiotensin–aldosterone system along with abnormalities in the renal tubules also play a part.
- Endothelial activation, dysfunction, and damage that are seen in hypertension are both a cause and effect of the raised blood pressure and contribute significantly to the maintenance of high blood pressure.

2.1 Introduction

Hypertension is often classified as 'primary' or 'essential' hypertension and 'secondary' hypertension. In secondary hypertension, often a well-defined cause is responsible for the raised blood pressure such as hyperaldosteronism or renal artery stenosis. Table 2.1 lists the common causes of secondary hypertension. However, in the vast majority of hypertensive patients, no obvious cause is found. In this chapter we will examine the different pathophysiological processes that are thought to cause the development and progression of high blood pressure. Blood pressure is directly proportional to the cardiac output/circulatory volume and the peripheral resistance. Each of these primary determinants is in turn determined by interaction of a complex series of factors which are depicted in Figure 2.1.

2.2 Increased circulating fluid volume (increased preload)

2.2.1 Sodium sensitivity and retention

Excess sodium intake and sodium sensitivity can cause hypertension by increasing fluid volume and preload, thereby increasing cardiac output as well as by effects on vascular reactivity and contractility. Hypertension is infrequent or almost absent in primitive communities with very low salt intakes, suggesting that a low-salt diet may protect against hypertension. However, in the Western world where practically everyone consumes a high-salt diet, only about one-third develop hypertension, suggesting a variable degree of blood pressure sensitivity to sodium. It is likely that the kidneys in susceptible individuals are unable to excrete an increased sodium load and therefore cause salt and water retention leading to increased circulating fluid volume and thereby to hypertension.

Table 2.1 Causes of secondary hypertension		
Renal	Endocrine	Other causes
• Renal parenchymal disease—glomerulo-nephritis • Polycystic kidneys • Diabetic nephropathy • Hydronephrosis • Renal artery stenosis • Renin-producing tumours • Renal tubular problems—Liddle's syndrome	• Acormegaly • Hypothyroidism • Hyperthyroidism • Cushing's syndrome • Hyperaldosteronism • Pheochromocytoma • Carcinoid • Exogenous source of increased estrogen, corticosteroids	• Acute stress • Arteriosclerosis • Paget's disease • Arteriovenous fistulae • Increased intracranial pressure

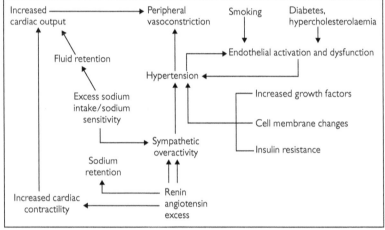

Figure 2.1 The various factors involved in the pathogenesis of hypertension and their complex interactions

2.2.2 **Resetting of the pressure-natriuresis feedback loop**

Pressure natriuresis is a phenomenon by which the kidneys excrete more salt and water when arterial pressure is raised. This is due to transmission of increased arterial pressure into peritubular capillaries, with a resultant increased hydrostatic pressure within the renal tubules and glomerulus, thereby reducing sodium and water reabsorption. This would cause the intravascular volume to reduce and return the capillary pressure and then the arterial pressure back to normal to close the negative feedback loop. A resetting of this feedback loop to accommodate higher pressures would lead to a failure of the kidneys to excrete increased amounts of sodium and water in the presence of an overload, and this could lead to the persistence of the increased circulatory volume and thence an increased pressure.

What causes this feedback loop to be reset is unclear. One of the explanations is that the constant increased sodium in the blood due to chronic increased ingestion could lead to a blunting of the response and the body readjusting itself to this chronic persistent increased load. Altered renal functions, changes in endothelial function, etc., may also contribute to this. A genetic predisposition, although not proved, could also be a likely explanation.

2.2.3 Nephron abnormalities

Nephron abnormalities such as presence of ischaemic nephrons that produce renin or a reduction in the number of nephrons with age decrease the ability to excrete sodium. Decreased filtration surface area due to conditions such as glomerular sclerosis also reduces the sodium excretion ability.

2.3 Renin–Angiotensin–Aldosterone System

The Renin–Angiotensin–Aldosterone System (RAAS) is one of the major players in the development of hypertension. The RAAS is responsible for the maintenance of normal body salt and water homeostasis. The multiple actions of angiotensin II act to minimize renal fluid and sodium losses and maintain blood pressure. This system is discussed in detail in the chapter on renovascular hypertension. Alterations in this system due to various conditions lead to the development of hypertension.

In hypertension, due to the increased perfusion pressures at the glomeruli, one would expect the plasma levels of renin to be low. However, the majority of patients with essential hypertension do not have low, suppressed plasma renin levels, but have 'inappropriately normal' or even elevated levels. This could be due to the presence of few ischaemic nephrons that produce increased levels of renin that mask the decreased renin secretion by the normal nephrons.

2.4 Hyperactive sympathetic nervous system

There is considerable evidence to suggest the presence of increased sympathetic nervous activity in early hypertension and in the offspring of hypertensive patients, a large number of whom will develop hypertension. In these patients there is a resetting of the arterial baroreceptors with resultant increase in sympathetic outflow from the vasomotor centre. This increased activity of the sympathetic nervous system will lead to peripheral vasoconstriction and thereby an increased blood pressure. This increase is further enhanced during physical emotional or mental stress. Stress elicits an increased cardiovascular reactivity to the increased sympathetic tone and over a prolonged period can lead to persistently high blood pressure.

2.5 Increased peripheral resistance

The final common feature of established hypertension is increased peripheral resistance. In the initial stages of hypertension, the increased perfusion pressures due to increased circulatory volumes can lead to a compensatory peripheral vasoconstriction. With time, this peripheral vasoconstriction can become permanent and will lead to the maintenance of hypertension. Changes in the endothelial function as in autocrine and paracrine factors also play a role in the persistence of this increased vascular tone.

2.6 Endothelial dysfunction

Hypertension is associated with endothelial activation and dysfunction. This is both a cause and an effect of the raised blood pressure. The endothelium may get activated due to various causes such as diabetes, smoking, hyperlipidaemia, etc., or the raised blood pressure itself. This activated endothelium then causes changes within itself that perpetuates the raised blood pressure.

One of the main features of this activated and later dysfunctional and damaged endothelium is the change to nitric oxide (NO). NO or endothelium-derived relaxing factor, as it was first called, is produced by the endothelium and helps reduce vascular tone. Damage to the endothelium results in decreased production of NO, resulting in decreased endothelium-dependent vasodilatation. This contributes to the maintenance of high blood pressure.

Oxidative stress, by the excess production of reactive oxygen species can also cause endothelial damage. Oxidative stress, which itself is caused by endothelial dysfunction, can then set up a vicious cycle which can lead to more damage and dysfunction. Oxidative stress can decrease the production of NO and can lead to the maintenance of the high blood pressure.

Other changes that occur in the endothelium with hypertension include increase in endothelins which are molecules produced by the endothelium that have profound vasoconstrictor effects. In addition, endothelins have positive inotropic and positive chronotropic effects on cardiomyocytes, proliferative effects on various cells, stimulation of hormone release, and modulation of central nervous activities. Bradykinins which are potent vasodilators are also decreased along with an increase in the levels of angiotensin-converting enzyme that is produced by the endothelium. The plasma concentration of kinins is however not high enough to affect blood pressure, but it is thought to act in a paracrine manner. Other vasodilators such as prostacyclins are also found to be decreased in hypertension.

2.7 **Insulin resistance**

The association between insulin resistance and hypertension is well established. There are many proposed mechanisms by which insulin resistance causes raised blood pressure and these include increased sympathetic nervous activity, increased renal sodium retention, and enhanced vascular hypertrophy. Of these, impaired vasodilatation may be particularly important. Although insulin increases sympathetic nervous activity to skeletal muscle, the effect is normally overridden by the direct vasodilatory effect of insulin. However, patients with hypertension may have a defect in this vasodilatory action, failing to increase muscle blood flow in response to insulin infusion.

2.8 **Other factors**

The natriuretic peptides (atrial, brain, and C-type natriuretic peptides, ANP, BNP, and CNP, respectively) are primarily made in the cardiac atria in response to atrial stretch and tend to cause salt and water excretion. Changes in these peptides have been demonstrated in hypertension. Similarly a role for argenine vasopressin (AVP) and adrenomedullin (a recently identified hormone) in the pathogenesis of hypertension has been suggested.

In addition to the above described mechanisms, it is important to note that genetic predisposition is a major factor. Environmental factors also play an important role such as the plasma calcium, diet, physical exercise, obesity, etc. Intrauterine influences may also play a part as it has been shown that babies with low birth weight are more likely to have higher blood pressures during adolescent life and hypertension during adult life. The exact mechanism involved here is not clear, but it is felt to be related to metabolic abnormalities that are seen in these babies such as insulin resistance, hyperlipidaemia, and diabetes.

Hypertension is also associated with a prothrombotic state and thrombotic events such as myocardial infarctions and thrombotic strokes, even though the blood vessels are subject to high pressures. This has been referred to as the 'thrombotic paradox of hypertension' or the 'Birmingham paradox'. The prothrombotic state occurs as hypertension fulfils Virchow's triad for thrombosis. We have changes in the vessel wall with the endothelial changes, and there are changes in the flow pattern of blood due to the high shear forces in hypertension; and third, there are changes in the blood constituents with platelet activation. This prothrombotic state should be kept in mind whilst managing a patient with hypertension.

In summary, the pathophysiology of hypertension is complex and multifactorial. There is no single cause that is identifiable, though abnormalities in the physiological mechanisms involved in maintaining normal blood pressure may play a part in its development. Hypertension is the net result of multiple complex factors that are interrelated and which then set up a vicious cycle of positive feedback.

Key references

Kearney PM, Whelton M, Reynolds K, *et al*. (2005). Global burden of hypertension: analysis of worldwide data. *Lancet*; 365: 217–23.

Lip GY (2003). Hypertension, platelets, and the endothelium: the 'thrombotic paradox' of hypertension (or 'Birmingham paradox') revisited. *Hypertension*; 41(2): 199–200.

Luke RG (1993). Essential hypertension: A renal disease? A review and update of the evidence. *Hypertension*, 21: 380–90.

Rodrigo R, Gonzalez J, Paoletto F (2011). The role of oxidative stress in the pathophysiology of hypertension. *Hypertension research*; 34:431–440.

Turnbull F (2003). Blood pressure lowering treatment trialists collaboration. Effects of different blood pressure lowering regimens on major cardiovascular events: results of prospectively designed overviews of randomized trials. *Lancet*; 362: 1527–45.

Chapter 3

Renovascular hypertension

Sunil Nadar

Key points

- Impaired renal flow due to obstruction of the renal arteries causes hypertension by activation of the renin–angiotensin–aldosterone system.
- The incidence of this disease is increasing due to the ageing population.
- Investigations to rule out renal artery stenosis should only be done in select patients where there is a clinical suspicion.
- Renal angiogram is the gold standard test for diagnosis.
- Medical therapy should be instigated in the first instance.
- Percutaneous angioplasty and surgical revascularization provide similar outcome results.

3.1 Introduction

Renovascular hypertension (RVHT) refers to hypertension that is caused by disease of renal perfusion, usually occlusive disease of these arteries. It was Goldblatt in 1934 who first demonstrated a relationship between renal perfusion and hypertension in mice. Subsequently, further studies in humans revealed the relationship between the kidneys and hypertension. RVHT is the clinical consequence of renin–angiotensin–aldosterone activation secondary to renal ischaemia. Renal ischaemia triggers the release of renin and a secondary elevation in blood pressure. Hyperreninaemia promotes conversion of angiotensin I to angiotensin II, causing severe vasoconstriction and aldosterone release.

3.2 Pathophysiology

Activation of the renin–angiotensin–aldosterone system (RAAS) is the main pathophysiological process in RVHT. In a normal kidney, any drop in the perfusion pressure in the kidney would activate the RAAS, causing salt and water retention and systemic vasoconstriction to help bring the blood pressure up. Also, the aldosterone produced by activation of the RAAS would cause efferent arteriolar constriction to increase perfusion pressure within the kidney. In the case of renal artery stenosis (RAS), the perfusion pressure within the kidneys is reduced. This causes activation of the RAAS in an attempt to increase renal perfusion, and thereby causes salt and water retention and systemic vasoconstriction. This is depicted in Figure 3.1.

The pathogenesis of RVHT also depends on whether the renal arterial occlusion is unilateral or bilateral. In the case of a unilateral RAS, the ischaemic kidney produces increased amounts of renin which produces increased aldosterone via angiotensin. However, in the presence of a normal contralateral kidney, the excess salt and water is excreted. However, the intense systemic vasoconstriction caused by the increased aldosterone keeps the blood pressure up.

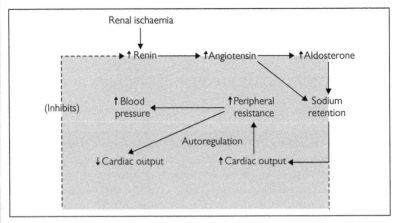

Figure 3.1 Pathophysiology of hypertension in renal artery stenosis

Conversely, in the absence of a normal kidney to excrete the excess stored salt and water, there is the added component of fluid overload which keeps the blood pressure up. However, in this situation the increased fluid load would cause some suppression of renin secretion.

The above changes depend on the time frame over which the renovascular occlusion takes place. If the renovascular occlusion is corrected, the processes are reversed and the blood pressure normalizes. However, if there is damage to renal parenchyma due to prolonged ischaemia, then the hypertension may be irreversible even with correction of the renal blood flow.

3.3 Aetiology

The aetiology of RAS and RVHT differs according to age and sex. Atherosclerotic disease affects mainly the proximal third of the main renal artery and is most common among older men. Fibromuscular dysplasia involves the distal two-thirds and branches of the renal arteries and is most common among younger women. Other clinical entities that may be associated with RVHT include acute arterial thrombosis or embolism, aortic dissection, arteriovenous malformation of the renal artery, and polyarteritis nodosa.

3.4 Incidence

The incidence of RVHT is less than 5% for the general population, but could be greater than 50% in hypertensive patients above the age of 70. It also appears to be more common among the white population than the black population. It is most common in younger women and older men with differing aetiologies as mentioned earlier. However, in view of the increasing age of the population, atherosclerotic RAS is becoming more common.

3.5 Clinical features

RVHT should be suspected in the following patients:

- Hypertensive patients with some renal impairment and modest proteinuria (levels < 1.5 g/d)
- Progressive renal insufficiency

- Refractory hypertension
- Accelerated or malignant hypertension
- Severe hypertension (diastolic blood pressure > 120 mmHg)
- Paradoxical worsening of hypertension with diuretic therapy or angiotensin-converting enzyme inhibitors (ACEI)
- Young patients
- Unprovoked hypokalaemia (serum potassium level < 3.6 mEq/L, often associated with metabolic alkalosis)
- Symptoms of atherosclerotic disease elsewhere in the presence of moderate-to-severe hypertension, particularly in patients older than 50 years
- Recurrent pulmonary edema in the setting of moderate-to-severe hypertension
- Presence of an unexplained atrophic kidney or asymmetric kidneys of greater than 1.5 cm difference
- Presence of an abdominal bruit (seen in around half of patients with RAS but also in around one-tenth of patients with essential hypertension, especially younger individuals).

3.6 **Investigations**

Investigating for RAS or RVHT in all patients with hypertension may not be practical or cost-effective. Patients with the features mentioned under the clinical findings may benefit from investigations to rule out RVHT.

3.6.1 **Lab tests**

Plasma renin activity

The baseline plasma renin activity (PRA) is elevated in 50–80% of patients with RVHT. However, this test is quite cumbersome and has yet to be standardized.

Renal vein renin measurements

Renal vein renin measurements compare renin release from each kidney and a 1.5-fold variation could suggest abnormal release from one kidney. False-negative and false-positive results are common.

3.6.2 **Imaging studies**

Magnetic resonance angiography has a sensitivity of 96–100% and a specificity of 71–96% for the detection of a main RAS of greater than 50%. Patient-specific problems such as claustrophobia and the presence of metallic implants and the cost and availability of the test would preclude the routine use of this test.

Spiral CT scan with angiography offers the diagnostic accuracy of arteriography and the lower risk of renal injury with IV digital subtraction angiography. It has a sensitivity and specificity of approximately 98% and 94%, respectively, for detecting significant RAS.

An intra-arterial digital subtraction angiogram (DSA) remains the gold standard among available tests for detecting RAS. It requires less radiopaque contrast than conventional angiography. A RAS of greater than or equal to 70% or a 50% stenosis with post-stenotic dilatation is considered hemodynamically significant.

Doppler ultrasonography provides both anatomic and functional assessment of the renal arteries. It has a sensitivity of 72–92% for the detection of RAS exceeding 70%. Both unilateral and bilateral disease can be picked up with this method. It can also be used to detect recurrent stenosis in patients previously treated with angioplasty or surgery. Difficulty in proper visualization and image acquisition is the main limitation of this test.

Radioisotope renogram has a high false-negative rate (20–25%), and is therefore not effective as a screening test. The predictive value, however, can be enhanced by the administration of captopril orally (25–50mg) 1 hour before the isotope is injected. Captopril inhibits the angiotensin II-mediated vasoconstriction and therefore leads to a decrease in renal perfusion in the kidney with the stenotic renal artery and causes a concurrent increase in renal perfusion in the normal kidney. This test would not yield a positive result in the case of bilateral RAS.

On assessing kidney size by ultrasound or intravenous pyelogram, the side with the RAS would have a smaller kidney. This test, however, has a low specificity.

3.7 Treatment

Once a haemodynamically significant lesion has been demonstrated, there are three options. Patients can continue on medical therapy or if that is not effective, they could be referred for relief of the obstruction either by percutaneous methods or by open surgical correction. However, it is recommended that medical therapy should be initiated in all patients in the first instance before referring for any surgical correction.

3.7.1 Medical care

All patients with RAS should be treated with antihypertensive drugs like any other hypertensive patient in the first instance. In the case of atherosclerotic RVHT, antilipid therapy may also be indicated. However, when the blood pressure proves difficult to control, surgical referral should be considered.

All classes of antihypertensive medications are used to treat RVHT. ACEIs would theoretically be the most useful drug in this situation as it would decrease the ischemia-induced rise in angiotensin production. However, in the case of unilateral RAS, this could cause deterioration in the perfusion in the affected kidney and a rise in serum markers of renal function. This deterioration in renal function may be reversible if noticed early. Not much is known about the use of angiotensin receptor blockers (ARBs) in this setting. Diuretics help in reducing the volume overload component of RVHT. Calcium-channel blockers (CCBs) may provide equally good control of hypertension, with presumably less impairment in function of the ischemic kidney than ACE inhibitors.

Aldosterone inhibitors such as spironolactone and eplerenone could also be used provided the renal functions are normal. Strict watch on serum potassium levels are mandatory especially when co-administered with drugs known to increase serum potassium (e.g. amiloride, triamterene, ACE inhibitors, angiotensin II inhibitors).

3.7.2 Surgical treatment

Relieving the obstruction could be undertaken either percutaneously or by open surgery. Percutaneous transluminal angioplasty (PTRA) is a non-surgical procedure used to open stenotic renal arteries, the most amenable lesions being those without total occlusion and those resulting from fibromuscular dysplasia. Outcomes appear to be significantly better than those associated with atherosclerotic stenosis, with cure reported in 8–20% of patients with atherosclerotic stenosis compared to 50–85% in those with fibromuscular lesions. Restenosis requiring repeat angioplasty was reported in fewer than 10% of patients with fibromuscular disease and in 8–30% of those with atherosclerotic stenosis. Improvement in blood pressure control with fewer antihypertensive medications was achieved in 30–35% and 50–60% of fibromuscular and atherosclerotic lesions, respectively.

Open surgical revascularization results in a cure rate of 80–90% of patients undergoing operation for focal atherosclerotic or fibromuscular RAS. The perioperative mortality rate is less than 5%. However, in patients with diffuse atherosclerosis, the complication rate with both surgery and angioplasty is relatively high.

The presence of renal failure poses not only additional risks, but also the potential for significant benefit. Studies have shown that those with renal failure at baseline had a higher mortality rate of around 25% within the next 2–3 years without revascularization. However, those patients whose renal functions improved after revascularization had significantly better survival rates.

Studies also do not show a benefit of angioplasty over surgery. However, angioplasty is the preferred first choice of procedure as it is non-invasive. Patients with fibroplastic disease do better than those with atherosclerotic disease whichever way they are treated, although those in the latter group would theoretically benefit from surgical revascularization due to the diffuse nature of the disease.

Key references

Aurell M, Jensen G (1997). Treatment of renovascular hypertension. *Nephron;* 75(4): 373–83.

Conlon PJ, O'Riordan E, Kalra PA (2000). New insights into the epidemio-logic and clinical manifestations of atherosclerotic renovascular disease. *American Journal of Kidney Disease;* Apr; 35(4): 573–87.

Safian RD and Textor SC (2001). Renal-artery stenosis. *New England Journal of Medicine;* Feb; 344(6): 431–42.

Textor S., Lerman L. (2011). State of the art: Renovascular hypertension and ischaemic nephropathy. *American Journal of hypertension;* 23: 1159.

Working Group on Renovascular Hypertension. (1987). Detection, evaluation, and treatment of reno-vascular hypertension. Final report. Working Group on Renovascular Hypertension. *Archives of Internal Medicine;* May; 147(5): 820–9.

Chapter 4

Primary hyperaldosteronism

Sunil Nadar

Key points

- Primary hyperaldosteronism is an important treatable cause of hypertension.
- It is caused by aldosterone-producing tumours.
- Screening would be beneficial in patients with resistant hypertension and young hypertensive patients.
- Serum potassium alone as a screening test for primary hyperaldosteronism would miss nearly two-thirds of patients.
- Ratio of plasma aldosterone to plasma renin activity is accepted as the test of choice for screening.
- Imaging tests help localize the tumour.
- Surgical removal of tumour should be the first choice of treatment if feasible.
- Spironolactone is the drug of choice for medical therapy if surgery fails or is not possible.

4.1 Introduction

Primary hyperaldosteronism (PHA) (also known as Conn's syndrome) is a condition in which an intra-adrenal abnormality leads to aldosterone production above the physiological requirements necessary to maintain normal electrolyte balance. This is in contrast to secondary hyperaldosteronism where extra-adrenal stimulatory factors, particularly renin excess, lead to aldosterone secretion above that required for maintaining normal electrolyte balance. The causes of primary hyperaldosteronism include aldosterone-producing adenoma, bilateral zona glomerulosa hyperplasia (ZGHP), glucocorticoid remediable hyperaldosteronism (GRA), idiopathic hyperaldosteronism, and rarely, adrenal carcinoma. It is estimated that the prevalence of this condition worldwide is around 1%.

4.2 Pathophysiology

The adrenal cortex can be divided into three distinct morphologic and functional zones. The outermost is the zona glomerulosa, which produces aldosterone; the middle zone is the zona fasiculata, which produces glucocorticoids; and the innermost is the zona reticularis, which produces the adrenal androgens.

Aldosterone, the major mineralocorticoid, is mainly concerned with salt and water homeostasis. Its secretion is pulsatile and is under the control of a wide variety of stimuli. The major controlling factor is the renin-angiotensin system, which in turn is activated by changes in fluid volume and sodium concentrations. When the receptors in the renal juxtaglomerular apparatus (JGA) detect sodium or water depletion, or low perfusion pressure, they activate renin release, which in turn breaks down renin substrate (angiotensinogen) to produce angiotensin 1. This hormone is almost inert but is rapidly converted to the active form—Angiotensin II—by the enzyme angiotensin-converting enzyme (ACE) in the vascular endothelium. Angiotensin II is a potent stimulus for aldosterone release, leading to sodium and water retention and potassium loss.

The production of excess aldosterone in PHA is partially autonomous and the sodium and water retention leads to suppression of plasma renin levels. Aldosterone secretion cannot be suppressed by volume expansion or increased sodium intake, as occurs in the normal population. The aldosterone excess can be partially suppressed by adrenocorticotropic hormone

Table 4.1 Causes of hyperaldosteronism and their distinguishing features				
Characteristic/ investigation	Aldosteronoma	Idiopathic (bilateral) hyperaldo-steronism	Unilateral or primary adrenal hyperplasia	Adrenal carcinoma
Age	Middle-aged; occasionally young, predominantly female	Older men	Middle-aged, occasionally young males or females	Middle-aged, occasionally young males or females
Serum potassium level	Moderately low	Mildly decreased	Mild to moderate decrease	Profound hypokalaemia
Urinary potassium levels	Mild to moderate increase	Mild increase	Mild to moderate increase	Very high
Plasma renin	Suppressed and very low	Moderately suppressed	Moderately to very suppressed	Moderately to very suppressed
Plasma or urinary aldosterone level	Moderately high	Lower than in aldosteronoma	Moderately increased	Very high
Plasma aldosterone response in postural test	Decreased or not increased in 70–80% of cases	Almost always increased	Decreased or not increased in 70–80% of cases	Often unchanged
Other features	Increased urinary 18-oxocortisol and 18-hydro-xycortisol; occasionally high level of cortisol production by the adenoma	Only aldoster-one and related corticosteroid produced in excess	Probably similar to idiopathic hyperaldosteronism	Often other cortico-steroids (androgen, oestrogen or cortisol) produced in excess
CT scan	Adenoma	Bilaterally enlarged glands or normal	Normal or unilateral enlargement	Large tumour
Scintigraphy	Increased uptake	Bilateral increased uptake	Limited data	Often no uptake; occasionally increased
Pathology	Solitary small adenoma	Macro-nodular or micro-nodu-lar hyperplasia	As in idiopathic	Large tumour with or without local invasion or metastasis

(ACTH) in most cases of aldosterone-producing adenoma, but appears in most patients to be unresponsive to angiotensin II. Table 4.1 gives the different causes of hyperaldosteronism and the differentiating features for each of them.

4.3 Clinical features

Conn originally described a patient with hypertension, hypokalaemia, and neuromuscular symptoms associated with an aldosterone-producing adrenal adenoma. These features still hold true, but they can be seen in many conditions with aldosterone excess and therefore are not specific to PHA. Aldosterone-producing adenomas occur more commonly in women than in men.

Some patients are asymptomatic, while others have symptoms related to hypertension (e.g. headache), hypokalaemia (polyuria, nocturia or muscle cramps), or both. Occasionally serious muscle weakness, paraesthesia, tetany, or paralysis resulting from profound hypokalaemia can be prominent, and such features may be more common in Asian patients. Severe retinopathy or malignant hypertension is uncommon.

4.4 Diagnosis

A high index of suspicion should be raised in patients with hypertension who have spontaneous diuretic-induced hypokalaemia, especially in the presence of a high sodium level. The other subgroups who merit investigation are patients resistant to therapy and young patients. It has been estimated that about 7.1% of patients with hypertension have biochemical results that indicate the need for investigations for PHA. Bendroflumethiazide and related thiazide diuretics in the low doses used nowadays usually do not cause hypokalaemia. Thus, a significant fall in potassium with thiazides may reflect underlying aldosterone excess.

Although spontaneous hypokalaemia in a patient with hypertension is a strong indicator that hyperaldosteronism is present, at least 20% of hypertensive patients have a low normal serum potassium level and this therefore is not useful as a diagnostic tool. Patients with hypertension of other aetiologies may also have a low serum potassium due to liquorice ingestion, diuretic, purgative abuse, etc. Therefore, a serum potassium level by itself would not be a good indicator of who needs further tests.

Box 4.1 summarizes the different tests that are useful in the diagnosis of PHA. Plasma renin activity is suppressed in patients with PHA, but a similar picture is seen in many patients with essential hypertension. In contrast, it is decreased in secondary hyperaldosteronism. The measurement of plasma renin activity has to be strictly standardized as it can vary with posture, time of day, and medications. Similarly, the measurement of a single value of plasma aldosterone has limited value as it varies considerably with posture, drugs, and time of day.

The ratio of plasma aldosterone-to-renin activity has been shown by many authors to be a more robust method of diagnosing PHA. However, due to the difficulties in checking these levels (it has to be standardized to the time of day, posture, etc.), it is not convenient or cost-effective to use as a screening method.

In addition to the screening tests mentioned earlier, further tests can be performed to determine the autonomy of aldosterone secretion by the adrenals and the more or less complete suppression of renin secretion. They involve measuring the levels of serum aldosterone with various stimuli such as saline infusions, or the administration of fludrocortisones, captopril or furosemide (Box 4.1). Lack of circadian variation of aldosterone secretion also helps diagnose PHA. Due to the availability of high-resolution imaging, most centres do not perform these dynamic tests, as most of them are cumbersome, and time consuming.

> ### Box 4.1 Tests for the diagnosis of primary hyperaldosteronism
>
> #### Screening tests
> - Serum potassium
> - Plasma renin activity
> - Plasma renin mass
> - Plasma aldosterone
> - Ratio of plasma aldosterone to renin
> - Urinary potassium levels
>
> #### Dynamic tests
> - Saline infusion test
> - Fludrocortisone suppression test
> - Captopril test
> - Combined stimulation by furosemide and posture
> - Response to infusion of potassium aspartate
> - Response to head-out full-body water immersion
>
> #### Tests to help localize the source of the extra hormone
> - Circadian rhythm of plasma aldosterone
> - Response to angiotensin II
> - Plasma 18-hydroxycorticosterone levels
> - Urinary 18-oxocortisol and 18-hydroxycortisol excretion
> - Imaging—CT, MRI.

Further tests such as plasma 18-hydroxycorticosterone and urinary 18-oxocortisol and 18-hydroxycortisol are required to distinguish the different types of primary hyperaldosteronism (Table 4.1).

Adrenal imaging is a very important tool in investigating hyperaldosteronism. Improved techniques of computed tomography (CT) scanning enable detection of adenomas of 10 mm or even 5 mm diameter. However, this test should be done only after the diagnosis of PHA has been firmly established biochemically to make sure that an 'incidentaloma' is not wrongly presumed to be an aldosterone-producing adenoma.

The adrenals can be imaged by either CT scanning or magnetic resonance imaging (MRI). The sensitivity and specificity of these techniques is, however, still not clear with different centres reporting different values. However, with the newer generation CT scanners, the image quality and the results of the two modalities should be comparable. Adrenal scintigraphy following the injection of radioiodine labelled 6-beta-iodomethylnorcholesterol and adrenal venous sampling also help localize tumours. The choice between the various tests depends entirely on the local experience and expertise.

4.5 **Pseudohyperaldosteronism**

These cases are characterized by hypertension with hypokalaemic alkalosis and suppressed unresponsive plasma renin activity to stimulating manoeuvres similar to classic hyperaldosteronism but the levels of plasma aldosterone are low. Some of the causes of pseudohyperaldosteronism include Liddle's syndrome, Cushing's syndrome, congenital adrenal hyperplasia with 11-beta-hydroxysteroid dehydrogenase deficiency, 17-alpha-hydroxysteroid dehydrogenase deficiency, and liquorice abuse. Although clinically it may be difficult to distinguish them from the syndromes of hyperaldosteronism, the low concentration of plasma aldosterone is the main feature of these pseudohyperaldosteronism syndromes.

4.6 **Recommendations for investigation**

Our recommendations for investigating a patient suspected of having PHA are summarized in Box 4.2. We would not recommend routine screening in all patients with hypertension. These patients should have a plasma aldosterone-to-renin ratio measured. A ratio of greater than 30 is taken as a cut-off for further investigations of hyperaldosteronism. These patients could then have further dynamic tests such as the captopril test or should go on directly to the imaging

---

Box 4.2 The subgroups of hypertensive patients in whom investigations for PHA are recommended

- Patients with resistant hypertension
- Those whose blood pressure is not controlled with three or more drugs
- Those with persistent hypokalaemia, either spontaneous or diuretic induced, especially in the presence of a high sodium level
- Relatively young patients (below the age of 40) even without any of the above factors

---

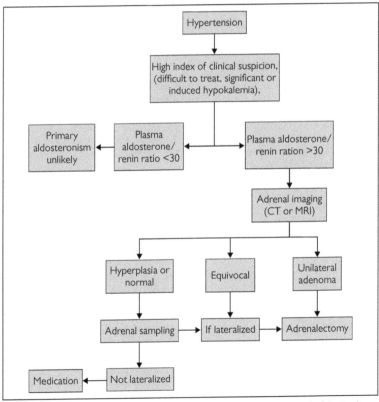

Figure 4.1 Algorithm for the management of a hypertensive patient suspected of having hyperaldosteronism

tests. Adrenal CT or MRI or an adrenal scintigraphy, depending upon the local expertise, is then recommended. If this shows a clear-cut adenoma, the patients could then be referred for surgery (Figure 4.1).

4.7 **Management**

4.7.1 **Medical**

The aldosterone antagonist spironolactone is the drug of choice and cornerstone of medical management. It can be started at 25 mg and increased up to 400 mg/day, either alone or with a loop diuretic. The level of hypertension and degree of hypokalaemia should be a guide.

It may take a few weeks before the blood pressure normalizes. If hypokalaemia is not a significant problem, a thiazide diuretic can be added at the start. Serum magnesium should also be monitored, as these patients tend to lose magnesium in the urine. Side effects such as painful gynaecomastia, nausea, fatigue, impotence, and profound hypokalaemia, especially when used with ACE inhibitors, can sometimes limit the use of spironolactone.

Eplerenone, a more selective aldosterone inhibitor, may also be used in patients not tolerant of spironolactone, as it has much fewer side effects. Alternatively, other potassium-sparing diuretics such as amiloride or triamterene may also be used. Amiloride is preferred because of its greater potency. Frequently other non-diuretic antihypertensives need to be added for adequate blood pressure control.

4.7.2 **Surgery**

Unilateral laparoscopic adrenalectomy is the procedure of choice for patients with aldosterone-producing adenomas. In patients with bilateral hyperplasia, asymmetrical aldosterone production, or primary adrenal hyperplasia, medical treatment with spironolactone is used as the treatment of choice.

In preparation for surgery, the serum potassium and blood pressure should be normalized, preferably with spironolactone or amiloride. Some patients in the post-operative period develop a salt-losing syndrome, possibly secondary to persistent suppression of the remaining normal adrenal gland. Some adrenal tumours produce sufficient cortisol to suppress ACTH and cortisol production in the contralateral adrenal gland. Thus, in the post-operative period, these patients may require glucocorticoid replacement therapy. In patients who are not suitable for surgery, arterial embolization of aldosteronoma with ethanol has also been reported.

4.8 **Conclusion**

PHA is an important cause of hypertension and it represents one of the few curable causes of hypertension. Although its true prevalence is debatable, it is estimated that up to 10% of patients with hypertension could have hyperaldosteronism. Care should also be taken to rule out other conditions, such as pseudohyperaldosteronism, which could mimic the findings of hyperaldosteronism.

In patients who do not seem to have any other risk factors, and especially in young patients with hypertensions, vigorous investigations must be undertaken to rule out this potentially treatable cause of hypertension. The results of surgery in a well-localized unilateral lesion are very successful and surgery should be offered to these patients. Medical management in those patients who do not fulfil criteria for surgery is fairly successful and should be optimized.

Key references

Blumenfeld JD, Sealey JE, Schlussel Y, *et al.* (1994). Diagnosis and treatment of primary hyperaldosteronism. *Annals of Internal Medicine;* 121(11): 877–85.

Bravo EL (1993). Primary hyperaldosteronism: new approaches to diagnosis and management. *Cleveland Clinic Journal of Medicine;* 60: 379–86.

Ferriss JB, Beevers DG, Brown JJ, *et al.* (1978). Clinical, biochemical and pathological features of low-renin ('primary') hyperaldosteronism. *American Heart Journal;* 95(3): 375–88.

Holland OB (1995). Primary hyperaldosteronism. *Seminars in Nephrology;* 15(2): 116–25.

Mattsson C, Young WF Jr. Primary aldosteronism: diagnostic and treatment strategies (2006). *Nature Clinical Practice Nephrology;* 2 (4):198

Russell RP, Masi AT, Ritcher ED (1972). Adrenal cortical adenomas and hypertension. *Medicine;* 51: 211–25.

Salomon MI and Tchertkoff V (1978). Incidence and role of adrenocortical tumors in hypertension. *Geriatrics;* 23(179): 184.

Weinberger MH, Grim CE, Hollifield JW (1979). Primary hyperaldosteronism; Diagnosis, localization and treatment. *Annals of Internal Medicine;* 67: 403–13.

Zavagli G, Ricci G, Gilli G, *et al.* (1999). An easy diagnostic approach to primary hyperaldosteronism. *Steroids;* 64: 296–300.

Chapter 5

Lifestyle influences on blood pressure

Kully Sandhu and Sunil Nadar

Key points

- Patient lifestyle choices affect patient blood pressure.
- Obesity and lack of physical exercise are major risk factors that can lead to hypertension.
- Excess alcohol can lead to hypertension.
- Stress has been associated with high blood pressure.
- Lifestyle changes are becoming recognized as important factors to treat hypertension.

5.1 Introduction

There are striking differences between different populations with regard to both incidence and prevalence of hypertension. It is well documented that industrialized nations have a higher prevalence of hypertension than the less developed nations. Although under reporting in the less developed nations may play a role in this difference, there are a number of studies to suggest that lifestyle has a bearing on blood pressure. This has led to recent national and international guidelines incorporating lifestyle modifications as first-line therapy and one that ought to be continued even if pharmacological therapy is required.

5.2 Obesity

Obesity is a growing problem, particularly in Europe and North America. This is not only confined to the native population; it also applies to migrants. Body mass index or BMI, is a commonly used index for assessing if an individual is obese and is the ratio weight in kilograms over square of height in meters. Several epidemiological studies have shown that BMI has a direct relationship to blood pressure—in other words, the higher the BMI the higher the blood pressure. CT studies suggest that increased visceral fat and upper body or central obesity have an association with hypertension. More recently the association with waist-to-hip ratio has a greater association with hypertension and other cardiovascular risk prediction than BMI. Maintenance of a healthy body weight (BMI of about 25 kg/m2) and waist circumference (102 cm for men and 88 cm for women) is recommended for non-hypertensive individuals to prevent hypertension and for hypertensive patients to reduce blood pressure (BP). The optimal BMI is unclear after results of two large meta-analyses of prospective observational population-based outcome studies. The Prospective Studies Collaboration concluded that mortality was lowest at a BMI of about 22.5–25 kg/m2, whereas a more recent meta-analysis concluded that mortality was lowest in overweight subjects.

The pathophysiological mechanism in which obesity causes hypertension is still not clearly understood. However, many studies seem to suggest that insulin resistance may play a pivotal role. Individuals with insulin resistance have a higher level of circulating insulin and this causes increased sympathetic nervous activity which results in not only vascular smooth-muscle proliferation but also increased sodium retention. A reduction of 10 lb (4.5 kg) may help reduce or even prevent hypertension. A reduction of approximately 20 lb (9 kg) may even reduce the blood pressure between 5–20 mmHg. Several studies have shown that a reduction in systolic and diastolic pressures occurs with weight loss. A meta-analysis of 11 studies showed that even a 1 kg reduction in body weight was associated with reduction of 1.6 mmHg and 1.3 mmHg in systolic and diastolic blood pressure. A Cochrane review of six randomized trials showed that a weight loss of 4–8% was associated with a 3 mmHg decrease in both systolic and diastolic blood pressures. In a meta-analysis, reductions of mean systolic and diastolic blood pressures of 4.4 mmHg and 3.6 mmHg respectively were associated with an average weight loss of 5.1 kg. Weight loss also appears to improve the efficacy of antihypertensive medication.

5.3. **Alcohol**

Many clinical and epidemiological studies have demonstrated the association between high alcohol intake and blood pressure. There are three cautions to be borne in mind when looking at alcohol consumption studies: the first is that many trials have not included patients who consume large quantity of alcohol; secondly, many patients tend to under-report the quantity of alcohol they consume; and thirdly, there is a complex pattern of type of alcohol consumed with different socioeconomic groups, therefore making analysis difficult. These variables are summarized in Box 5.1. However, consumption of 80 g per day has been associated with raised blood pressure, especially in hypertensive patients. Blood pressure also decreases when alcohol consumption is stopped or reduced and importantly it remains low in abstinence.

A systematic review of meta-analysis studies has shown alcohol restriction reduces both systolic and diastolic blood pressure by 2.7 mmHg and 1.4 mmHg respectively. Excess alcohol consumption is also associated with atrial fibrillation and cardiomyopathy. Therefore one can ask how much alcohol consumption is safe? Currently there are conflicting data. Interestingly, the Physicians Health Study cohort reported that patients who consumed alcohol daily, weekly, or even monthly had lower reduced total and cardiovascular mortality than patients who rarely consumed alcohol or consumed none at all. This 'beneficial' effect of low to moderate alcohol consumption was seen in patients regardless of whether they had a blood pressure of

Box 5.1 Factors affecting the effect of alcohol on blood pressure
Age
Sex
Ethnicity
Amount of alcohol
Duration of alcohol consumption
Type of beverage
Drinking habit such as binge drinking
Obesity
Concomitant cigarette smoking
Level of physical exercise
Physiological stress

Table 5.1 Cross-sectional studies investigating the association between alcohol consumption and hypertension

Authors (year)	Findings
Kaiser-Permanente Multiphasic Health Examination study 1977	Of the cohort of 83 947 subjects, men who drank six or more drinks per day had a mean blood pressure that was 10.9 mmHg higher than those who were non-drinkers
Framingham study 1983	Of the cohort of 5209 subjects, heavy drinkers were twice as likely to have hypertension
INTERSALT study, 1994	In the cohort of 4626 men and 4647 women aged between 20 and 59, men who drank 300–499 ml of alcohol per week had average blood pressures that were 2.7 mmHg systolic and 1.6 mmHg diastolic higher than non-drinkers

140/90 mmHg or less. The study also reported that consumption of a single alcoholic drink once a month could reduce overall cardiovascular mortality by 18%.

The Seventh Report of the Joint National Committee on the prevention, detection, evaluation, and treatment of high blood pressure (JNC-7) recommended no more than two alcoholic drinks per day for men and one per day for women or men of lighter build. The Fourth British Hypertension Society Report (BHS-IV) recommends not more than three units a day for men and two units a day for women as primary prevention of hypertension, and in established hypertensives, no more than 21 units a week for men and 14 units a week for women. (A unit of alcohol is around is 10 ml of absolute alcohol, which is equivalent to 95 ml of wine, a half-pint of beer, or a single pub measure of 25 ml serving of spirits) Abiding by these limits could reduce blood pressures by 2–4 mmHg. These seem to suggest that mild to moderate alcohol consumption may be of some benefit, but moving to moderate to severe consumption is associated with higher blood pressure and increased risk of stroke.

There have been many cross-sectional population studies that have investigated the association between alcohol and hypertension (Table 5.1). Prospective studies (Table 5.2) such

Table 5.2 Prospective studies demonstrating the link between alcohol consumption and hypertension

Authors	Patient population	Findings
Chicago Peoples Gas Company study 1981	1899 White male employees	At baseline, the 'problem drinkers' had a higher incidence of high blood pressure (> 160mm Hg systolic and > 95 mmHg diastolic). At four-years follow-up, the problem drinkers had an even greater increase in blood pressure than the non-problem drinkers
The Chicago Western Electric Company study 1981	1899 White male employees	Men who consumed more than six drinks a day had a higher baseline blood pressure which significantly increased after four-years follow-up
The American Nurses study 1990	58 218 nurses were followed up for four years	Those drinking more than 20 g of alcohol per day had a significantly increased risk of hypertension which was dose-dependent
Nakayama et al. 1973	Hospitalized men were followed up over a period of 2–11 years	The blood pressure at follow-up was related with the baseline alcohol consumption
Framingham study 1983		Those with increased alcohol consumption were more likely to have higher blood pressure

as those in the Chicago Peoples Gas Company and the Chicago Western Electric Company confirm what the cross-sectional studies indicated. Interventional studies have also conclusively demonstrated a direct relationship between alcohol consumption and blood pressure. In these studies, blood pressure reduction was demonstrated in subjects with increased alcohol intake (> 80 g day) who abstained during their stay in hospital.

The relationship between alcohol consumption and blood pressure appears to be a complex one that has not as yet been fully elucidated. Many factors appear to affect the relationship between alcohol and raised blood pressure, summarized in Box 5.1. The amount of alcohol consumed, duration of consumption, and variability of consumption (e.g. binge drinking) appeared to be important factors. Those with low variability of alcohol consumption had lower blood pressures. The exact mechanism by which alcohol causes hypertension is not clear.

Stimulation and intense catecholamine release is thought to be a major contributor to raised blood pressure. Some authors suggest the presence of 'episodic withdrawal' in between episodes of alcohol consumption in heavy drinkers, which leads to this sympathetic stimulation. Other mechanisms described include an increase in plasma cortisol levels, increased vascular sensitivity, and endothelial dysfunction. Some suggest a genetic predisposition.

5.4 Physical activity

Observational cross-sectional studies have shown that people with a regular regime of physical activity have blood pressure levels about 5 mmHg lower than inactive subjects. A meta-analysis of 29 randomized controlled trials of aerobic exercise training programs of four weeks or more including both men and women has shown that exercise training reduced systolic blood pressure by 4.7 mmHg and diastolic blood pressure by 3.1 mmHg. The Hypertension Prevention Trial noted a 4% reduction in body weight over three years was associated with a 2.4/1.8 mmHg reduction in systolic and diastolic blood pressure. Exercise helps to reduce weight, increase insulin sensitivity, and improves overall 'well-being'.

Physical activity has an important influence on blood pressure and overall cardiovascular disease risk. Many clinical trials have demonstrated that increasing physical exercise can reduce blood pressure. Although no exercise regime is currently rated to be better than another, most exercise regimens tested have been aerobic exercise, defined as rhythmic exercise that involves large muscle movements (running, cycling, walking, or swimming) and that causes increases in heart rates. Meta-analysis has found that physical activity reduces both systolic and diastolic blood pressure in all population groups; the only exception was diastolic blood pressure in older patients. Reduction of blood pressure was also seen in normotensive patients. Dynamic exercises, such as weight training, has not been shown to decrease blood pressure or cardiovascular disease. The beneficial effects of exercise appear to plateau with the maximum benefit achieved by exercising three times per week. This is reflected in current guidelines that advocate moderate intensity for at least 30 minutes at least three times per week. Moderate-intensity exercise is that which causes the heart rate to rise to 50–70% of the maximum age predicted heart rate (which is calculated by subtracting age from 220). The importance of finding an activity that patients enjoy is of vital importance to maintain adherence.

5.5 Psychological stress and anxiety

Psychological factors play an important part in an individual's overall well-being. A major psychological component includes what is broadly referred to as 'stress'. The word 'stress' has various connotations, is used in a number of ways, and could mean different things in different situations. Psychological stress may result from any number of causes such as personal relationship, socio-economic, and employment stresses, and studies have shown higher incidence of blood pressure in patients who reported to be suffering from stress. Stressful situations leading to a heightened sympathetic drive with consequent increased catecholamine release have often been implicated as the aetiology of increased blood pressure in such patients. Meditation includes a variety of techniques; for example, repetition of a word or phrases, specific body movement and postures with careful attention to breathing patterns all appear to help the patient achieve a state of inner calm, detachment, and focus. Meditation has been shown to reduce blood pressure in one well-designed study that addressed baseline blood pressure measurements adequately, although other studies have been inconsistent. Long-term follow-up of 202 patients in two small studies indicated that transcendental meditation may even reduce mortality in patients with hypertension. Meditation may have other benefits and does not appear to be harmful except in patients with psychosis.

5.6 Smoking

Smoking is a well-recognized risk factor for cardiovascular disease. However, more recently smoking has been demonstrated to have a pressor effect that can raise ambulatory daytime blood pressure. Nicotine in cigarettes is believed to stimulate the sympathetic drive and in doing so causes release of adrenaline and noradrenaline. In fact, smoking has been associated with a 4 mmHg and 3 mmHg rise in systolic and diastolic blood pressure when compared with a placebo. Hypertensive patients who smoked had more frequent cardiovascular events than hypertensive non-smokers. Studies have also shown that hypertensive males who smoke not only had greater incidence of both ischaemic and haemorrhagic stroke but also the risk was related to the number of cigarettes smoked. Smoking cessation is an imperative and integral part of any lifestyle modification designed to reduce hypertension and cardiovascular disease

5.7 Dietary patterns

Diet is one of the main distinguishing factors of any given community and therefore it could well have a bearing on the different blood pressure profiles.

Fruits and vegetables. Studies have shown that a predominantly vegetarian diet is often present in those cultures that have generally low blood pressure. Similarly in industrialized nations, vegetarians have lower average blood pressure levels than comparable non-vegetarian populations. The so-called Mediterranean diet, rich in fruits and vegetables, has been shown to be associated with lower blood pressures. Indeed, such diets when introduced in studies (the Dietary Approaches to Stop Hypertension or DASH study) appeared to reduce blood pressure by almost the same amount as a single antihypertensive agent.

Potassium. The International Study of Salt and Blood pressure (INTERSALT) demonstrated an association of higher levels of urinary potassium excretion with lower blood pressures. Diets rich in fruits and vegetables have a high potassium content, which could explain the benefit of these kinds of diets. The exact mechanism of action is not clear but it is likely that increased potassium intake affects sodium excretion and could lead to changes in intravascular volume.

Sodium. There is considerable amount of evidence, both from animal experiment studies and from clinical trials and epidemiologic studies, that increased sodium intake increases blood pressure. An increased intake of potassium tends to offset this effect of sodium on blood pressure to a great extent. The INTERSALT study which investigated the relation of sodium to blood pressure included over 10 000 men and women from over 32 countries. It found a highly significant relationship between sodium intake and blood pressure, and mean blood pressure was lower by 10/6 mmHg in those whose sodium intake is lower by 100 mmol/day. The exact mechanism is not clear but it is likely that increased sodium intake causes more fluid retention and thereby increases blood pressure by a volume overload.

Key references

Chobanian AV, Bakris GL, Black HR, et al. (2003). Seventh report of the Joint National Committee on Prevention, Detection, Evaluation, and Treatment of High Blood Pressure. *Hypertension*; 42: 1206–52.

Flegal KM, Kit BK, Orpana H, et al. (2013). Association of all-cause mortality with overweight and obesity using standard body mass index categories. A systematic review and meta-analysis. *JAMA*; 309: 71–82.

Jordana J, Yumukb V, Schlaich M, et al. (2012) Joint statement of the European Association for the Study of Obesity and the European Society of Hypertension: obesity and difficult to treat arterial hypertension. *Journal of Hypertension*; 30: 1047–55.

Kawano Y, Abe H, Takishita S, et al. (1998). Effects of alcohol restriction on 24-hour ambulatory blood pressure in Japanese men with hypertension. *American Journal of Medicine*; 105(4): 307–11.

Kurth T, Kase CS, Berger K, et al. (2003) Smoking and the risk of hemorrhagic stroke in men. *Stroke*; 34: 1151–55.

Norris SL, Zhang X, Avenell A, et al. (2005). Long-term non pharmacological weight loss interventions for adults with pre-diabetes. *Cochrane Database Systematic Reviews*; CD005270.

Prospective Studies Collaboration (2009). Body-mass index and cause-specific mortality in 900 000 adults: collaborative analyses of 57 prospective studies. *Lancet*; 373: 1083–96.

Shaw K, Gennat H, O'Rourke P, et al. (2006). Exercise for overweight or obesity. *Cochrane Database Systematic Reviews*; CD003817.

The Task Force for the management of arterial hypertension of the European Society of Hypertension (ESH) and of the European Society of Cardiology (ESC) (2013). 2013 ESH/ESC Guidelines for the management of arterial hypertension *European Heart Journal*; 34, 2159–219

Whelton SP, Chin A, Xin X, et al. (2002). Effect of aerobic exercise on blood pressure: a meta-analysis of randomized, controlled trials. *Annals of Internal Medicine*; 136: 493–503.

Xin X, He J, Frontini MG, et al. (2001). Effects of alcohol reduction on blood pressure: a meta-analysis of randomized controlled trials. *Hypertension*; 38: 1112–27.

Yamagishi K, Iso H, Kitamura A, et al. (2003). Smoking raises the risk of total and ischemic strokes in hypertensive men. *Hypertension Research*; 26: 209–17.

Chapter 6

Diagnosis and investigations of hypertension

Sunil Nadar

> ### Key points
>
> - The diagnosis of hypertension should not be made based on a single elevated office blood pressure reading.
> - Ambulatory blood pressure monitoring will help in making the diagnosis of true hypertension and rule out 'white coat hypertension'.
> - The investigations for hypertension include evaluation of the presence of target organ damage to rule out causes of secondary hypertension.
> - Tests for secondary hypertension should only be done in the case of a strong clinical suspicion.
> - Assessment of a patient with hypertension should include overall assessment of risk of cardiovascular disease.

6.1 Introduction

Hypertension as a risk factor for cardiovascular disease has been proved without doubt. However, there is still some debate regarding the levels of blood pressure that separate abnormal blood pressure (hypertension) from normal pressure and what level of blood pressure constitutes hypertension. However, as it is a continuous variable, there should not be a precise cut-off value. Similarly, in terms of cardiovascular risk, the presence of other co-existent risk factors may increase risk in a particular individual in spite of comparatively low blood pressure. The presence of hypertension could also be defined pragmatically as that level of blood pressure which needs to be reduced in order to prevent cardiovascular and cerebrovascular events.

6.2 Blood pressure criteria

The seventh Joint National Committee on detection, evaluation, and treatment of high blood pressure (JNC-7) provides a widely accepted classification. The European Society of Hypertension (ESH) and the British Hypertension Society (BHS) have provided a modified version of this, which is also globally accepted. These have been compared in Table 6.1. The latest guidelines by the ESH (2013) have not changed the previous classifications of hypertension as described by them previously in 2007 and 2003.

What is significant with the classification is the class of 'prehypertension' that has been added to the JNC-7 guidelines. This group has been added in response to new epidemiological data that suggest that those who previously fell into the category of 'high normal' had a higher chance of developing hypertension with increasing age. The JNC-7 guidelines emphasize that they do not consider it a disease category; rather, they wish to identify individuals at high risk

Table 6.1 Classification of hypertension based on the British Hypertension Society and European Society of Hypertension guidelines

Category	Systolic blood pressure (mmHg)	Diastolic blood pressure (mmHg)	JNC-7 classification
Optimal	< 120	< 80	Normal
Normal	< 130	< 85	Prehypertension
High normal	130–139	85–89	Prehypertension
Grade 1 hypertension (mild)	140–159	90–99	Stage 1 hypertension
Grade 2 hypertension (moderate)	160–179	100–109	Stage 2 hypertension
Grade 3 hypertension (severe)	> 180	> 110	Stage 2 hypertension
Isolated systolic hypertension Grade 1	140–159	< 90	
Isolated systolic hypertension Grade 2	> 160	< 90	

JNC-7: Seventh Joint National committee on detection, evaluation, and treatment of high blood pressure.

of developing hypertension so that both the individuals and their treating physicians will be encouraged to intervene to prevent or delay the onset of hypertension. The JNC-7 report does not recommend the use of medication for this group, but instead recommends the initiation of a strict lifestyle modification programme.

6.3 **Measurement of blood pressure**

As the level of blood pressure is the basis of the diagnosis of hypertension, it is very important that blood pressure is measured in a standardized way. Box 6.1 and Table 6.2 give accepted guidelines regarding this.

There are various factors that affect the measurement of blood pressure. These include the following:

- Time of day—due to the diurnal variation of blood pressure
- Setting—blood pressure readings in the hospital setting tend to be higher especially when taken by a physician rather than a nurse
- Environmental—the room temperature can affect the readings
- In case of the manual sphygmomanometers—loud ambient noise can impair hearing the Korotkoff sounds properly
- Rapid deflation of the cuff
- Recent caffeine ingestion or cigarette smoking
- Recent alcohol consumption
- Recent physical exertion (including rushing to reach the clinic, etc.)
- Stress (e.g. driving to reach the clinic and inability to find parking space, etc.).

Many factors affect the accurate recording of blood pressure and therefore great care must be adopted before labelling a person as a hypertensive. Single office blood pressure readings are

Box 6.1 Ideal measurement of blood pressure

Patient conditions
- Sit quietly for at least five minutes with the arm bared and supported at the level of the heart and the back resting against a chair
- No caffeine or smoking within 30 minutes of testing

Equipment
- Well-calibrated machine
- Cuff should encircle at least 80% of the circumference of arm and cover two-thirds of the length of the arm (small bladder can cause false high readings).

Technique
- Bell of stethoscope should be used
- Avoid excess pressure
- At least two readings five minutes apart per examination
- Three sets of readings one week apart
- Cuff should be raised at least 20 mmHg above the disappearance of the radial pulse
- Cuff should be deflated by 3 mmHg/second
- Record phase V of the Korotkoff sounds—disappearance of the sounds (except in children where phase IV or muffling of the sounds is preferable)

Table 6.2 Recommended cuff size

	Bladder width × length (cm)	Arm circumference (cm)
Small adult/child	12 × 18	< 23
Standard adult	12 × 26	< 33
Large adult	12 × 40	< 50
Adult thigh	20 × 42	< 53

not sufficient to make the diagnosis of hypertension. Multiple high readings and even the use of ambulatory blood pressure monitoring may be required to make a definitive diagnosis of hypertension and start the patient on life-long therapy.

Diurnal variation is seen in blood pressure readings. The blood pressure often drops substantially during the night. The nocturnal blood pressures can fall by up to 15% of the daytime values. This is due to the diurnal variations in the secretions of different hormones, especially the steroid hormones, and a decrease in sympathetic activity. It is also thought to be due to the result of sleep and inactivity, as patients who are bed-bound do not have such substantial night-time falls in blood pressure but can have very modest falls of up to 5%.

Individuals whose blood pressure recordings do not show this night-time fall are called 'non-dippers' and those who do have this night-time 'dip' in blood pressure are referred to as 'dippers'. The following factors are associated with 'non-dipping':

- Old age
- Cognitive dysfunction
- Diabetes
- Obesity

- Endothelial dysfunction
- Renal dysfunction
- Left ventricular hypertrophy

'Non-dippers' are considered to be at higher risk of cardiovascular events. It has been demonstrated by some studies that those who 'dip' excessively, especially in the presence of left ventricular hypertrophy, are also at a higher risk of excess cardiovascular events.

6.4 White-coat hypertension

This refers to the condition where the blood pressure taken in a hospital or clinic setting is high (within the hypertensive range of > 140/90 mmHg)) whilst the blood pressure in an out-of-office setting is below 135/85 mmHg. As mentioned earlier, most patients have a higher reading taken in the office setting, including patients with hypertension—this is referred to as the 'white-coat effect'. However, in those individuals with white-coat hypertension, the blood pressure returns to normal limits when they are out of the office setting.

The recognition of white-coat hypertension is important as it precludes the need for antihypertensive treatment in these patients. There is, however, some debate regarding the prognosis and the cardiovascular risk of these patients with conflicting data available. The major determinant of prognosis is the presence of other cardiovascular risk factors such as diabetes, obesity, smoking, etc. These patients should therefore be monitored and counselled regarding lifestyle modifications.

6.5 Ambulatory blood pressure monitoring

This involves a recording of the blood pressure by means of a calibrated machine that automatically records the blood pressure over 24 hours whilst the individual carries out their normal daily routine. The machine can be set to take readings at regular intervals every 15–60 minutes during the day and generally just once every two hours during the night. This is useful to rule out a 'white-coat effect' in patients with 'difficult-to-treat' hypertension and in patients who do not have hypertension. It is also useful to check efficacy of therapy and to identify 'dippers' and 'non-dippers'. In addition, studies have demonstrated that target organ damage such as left ventricular hypertrophy and increased carotid intima-media thickness correlate more with the ambulatory blood pressure (ABP) readings than office readings. ABP readings have also been shown in a meta-analysis to be a more sensitive predictor of cardiovascular risk than office readings.

6.6 Clinical assessment of patients with hypertension

Once the diagnosis of hypertension is made, a full clinical examination must occur to look for any cause of secondary hypertension. An assessment must also be made to seek evidence of target organ damage. This involves the following:

- Examination of the retina—to rule out hypertensive retinopathy
- Checking blood pressure in both arms and in the lower limbs and looking for radio-femoral delay or radio-radial delay to rule out coarctation of aorta
- Listening for renal artery bruits
- Palpation for any abdominal renal mass

> ## Box 6.2 Investigations for secondary hypertension
>
> **Hormone assays**
> - Cortisol levels
> - Urinary metanephrines
> - Urinary corticosteroid levels
> - Urinary vanyl-mandelic acid
> - Plasma renin activity
>
> **Imaging tests**
> - Echocardiogram
> - Ultrasound renal tract and adrenals
> - Computed tomography of kidneys and adrenals
> - Doppler ultrasound of the renal arteries
> - Renal angiogram
> - Magnetic resonance imaging of adrenals

- Electrocardiogram or echocardiogram to look for left ventricular hypertrophy and atrial fibrillation
- Urinalysis for proteinuria

6.7 Investigations

The investigations for a patient diagnosed with hypertension follow the same principles as that for clinical examination in these patients. It is to look for evidence of target organ damage and also to rule out secondary causes of hypertension.

Initial laboratory tests include the following:

- Electocardiogram
- Echocardiogram
- Urinalysis for proteinuria
- Blood urea and electrolytes

Tests for secondary hypertension should be done only if there is a strong clinical suspicion such as in young patients, patients with uncontrollable hypertension, or those with malignant hypertension. All guidelines suggest that routine screening of all patients with hypertension for secondary causes is not a cost-effective form of management as these constitute only a small percentage of the entire hypertensive population. The details of the different tests (Box 6.2) will be discussed in the specific chapters.

6.8 Assessing cardiovascular risk

The relationship between blood pressure and risk of cardiovascular events is continuous, consistent, and independent of other risk factors. The higher the blood pressure, the greater the chance of heart attack, heart failure, stroke, and kidney diseases. The easy and rapid calculation of a Framingham coronary heart disease (CHD) risk score (Tables 6.3 and 6.4) or the joint British Societies cardiovascular disease risk prediction charts may assist the clinician and patient in demonstrating the benefits of treatment. Management of these other risk factors is essential

Table 6.3 Calculation of Framingham risk score for men

Age	Points	Total cholestrol	Points at ages 20–39	Points at ages 40–49	Points at ages 50–59	Points at ages 60–69	Points at ages 70–79
20–34	−9	< 160	0	0	0	0	0
35–39	−4	160–199	4	3	2	1	0
40–44	0	200–239	7	5	3	1	0
45–49	3	240–279	9	6	4	2	1
50–54	6	≥ 280	11	8	5	3	1
55–59	8						
60–64	10		Points at ages 20–39	Points at ages 40–49	Points at ages 50–59	Points at ages 60–69	Points at ages 70–79
65–69	11						
70–74	12						
75–79	13	Non-smoker	0	0	0	0	0
		Smoker	8	5	3	1	1

HDL	Points	Systolic BP	If untreated	If treated
≥ 60	−1	< 120	0	0
50–59	0	120–129	0	1
40–49	1	130–139	1	2
< 40	2	140–159	1	2
		≥ 160	2	3

Points total	10-year risk	Points total	10-year risk
< 0	< 1%	11	8%
0	1%	12	10%
1	1%	13	12%
2	1%	14	16%
3	1%	15	20%
4	1%	16	25%
5	2%	≥ 17	≥ 30%
6	2%		
7	3%		
8	4%		
9	5%		
10	6%		

Table 6.4 Calculation of Framingham risk score for women						
Age	points	Total cholestrol	Points at ages 20–39	Points at ages 40–49	Points at ages 50–59	Points at ages 60–69	Points at ages 70–79
20–34	−7	< 160	0	0	0	0	0
35–39	−3	160–199	4	3	2	1	1
40–44	0	200–239	8	6	4	2	1
45–49	3	240–279	11	8	5	3	2
50–54	6	≥ 280	13	10	7	4	2
55–59	8						
60–64	10		Points at ages 20–39	Points at ages 40–49	Points at ages 50–59	Points at ages 60–69	Points at ages 70–79
65–69	11						
70–74	14						
75–79	16	Non-smoker	0	0	0	0	0
		Smoker	9	7	4	2	1

HDL	Points	Systolic BP	If untreated	If treated
≥ 60	−1	< 120	0	0
50–59	0	120–129	1	3
40–49	1	130–139	2	4
< 40	2	140–159	3	5
		≥ 160	4	6

Points total	10-year risk	Points total	10-year risk
<9	<1%	20	11%
9	1%	21	14%
10	1%	22	17%
11	1%	23	22%
12	1%	24	27%
13	2%	≥ 25	≥ 30%
14	2%		
15	3%		
16	4%		
17	5%		
18	6%		
19	8%		

and should follow the established guidelines for controlling these co-existing problems that contribute to overall cardiovascular risk.

Key references

National high blood pressure education coordinating committee (1990). National high blood pressure education programme working group report on ambulatory blood pressure monitoring. *Archives of Internal Medicine*; 150: 2270–80.

Chobanian AV, Bakris GL, Black HR, *et al.* (2003). National Heart, Lung, and Blood Institute Joint National Committee on Prevention, Detection, Evaluation and Treatment of High Blood Pressure; National High Blood Pressure Education Program Coordinating Committee. *Hypertension*; 42:1206–52

Williams B, Poulter N, Brown MJ, *et al.* (2004). British hypertension society guidelines for hypertension management 2004 (BHS-IV); Summary, *British Medical Journal*; 328: 634–40.

The Task Force for the management of arterial hypertension of the European Society of Hypertension (ESH) and of the European Societyof Cardiology (ESC)(2013). 2013 ESH/ESC Guidelines for the management of arterial hypertension. *European Heart Journal*; 34, 2159–230230

Part 2

Complications of hypertension

Chapter 7

Hypertension: a cardiovascular risk factor

Rajesh Nambiar

Key points

- Hypertension is a strong risk factor for cardiovascular disease.
- Hypertension usually occurs in the presence of other cardiovascular risk factors.
- The treatment of hypertension leads to a reduction in future cardiovascular risk.

7.1 Introduction

Hypertension is a common and independent risk factor for the development of coronary artery disease, cerebrovascular disease, peripheral artery disease, and heart failure. Hypertension plays a vital role the development and progression of atherosclerotic vascular disease. It increases the risk by two- to three3 fold by accelerated atherosclerosis. The correlation between cerebrovascular disease and hypertension is derived from the long-term prospective epidemiologic data from the Framingham Heart Study.

7.2 Magnitude of the problem

Despite early detection, evaluation, and the initiation of early therapy, the prevalence and incidence of hypertension remains high. Hypertension is the largest risk factor burden for cardiovascular disease and it is growing in prevalence and is poorly controlled. As Laws and colleagues stated, 'overall about 80% of the attributable burden of hypertension occurs in low income and middle income economies'. The prevalence of hypertension in the United States has increased from 24.4% in 1990 to 28.9% in 2004. This has been attributed to the population becoming older and obese. Prevalence of hypertension increases with age and is higher in the black population than in the white population. Interestingly, it has also been shown that the mortality rate for coronary heart disease was lower in black men with a diastolic pressure exceeding 90 mmHg than in white men, but the mortality rate for cerebrovascular disease was higher. Hypertension rates in US Hispanics of Mexican origin are lower than those in whites. The Prospective Studies Collaborative found that the age specific associations of ischaemic heart disease (IHD) mortality with blood pressure (BP) to be slightly greater for women than for men, and concluded that 'for vascular mortality, sex is of little relevance'. In the US, women have a higher prevalence of systolic BP greater than 140.

Table 7.1 Number of other cardiovascular risk factors in hypertensive patients aged 18–65 in the Framingham Heart Study

Number of risk factors	% with risk factors	
	Men	Women
0	24.4	19.5
1	29.1	28.1
2 or more	46.5	52.4

7.3 **Hypertension and other cardiovascular risk factors**

Hypertension tends to occur in association with other metabolic risk factors like dyslipidemia, impaired glucose tolerance, abdominal obesity, hyperinsulinemia, and hyperuricemia. Hypertension as an isolated risk factor occurs in less than 20% of the general population. Approximately 60% of the hypertensive patients in the Framingham Heart Study had two or more risk factors (Table 7.1). An increase in cardiovascular death is related to the association of hypertension and these risk factors. The causes of metabolic clustering of hypertension with dyslipidemia, impaired glucose tolerance, hyperinsulinemia, obesity, and left ventricular hypertrophy (LVH) include insulin resistance and sympathetic overdrive. In the Framingham Heart Study, the risk factors that were associated with hypertension were predominantly obesity and weight gain on follow-up. A 30% increase in atherogenic risk factor clustering was noted with a 2.25 kg weight gain.

7.4 **Cardiovascular hazards**

Hypertension predisposes the individual to develop coronary artery disease, stroke, and peripheral artery disease. Clinical sequelae of hypertension shows a two- to fourfold increase as compared to a normotensive individual of the same age. The risk ratio is the highest for heart failure and stroke; however, coronary heart disease is the most common hazard for hypertension because of the higher incidence in the general population.

Hypertension plays an important role in atherogenesis, hence lowering the BP may prevent or slow down atherosclerosis in predisposed vascular beds. Risk of cardiovascular diseases increases with incremental rise in blood pressure. Between the ages of 40 and 70, a two-fold increase in the risk of cardiovascular disease is noted with 20 mmHg of systolic BP or 10 mmHg of diastolic blood pressure.

High normal BP (130–139/85–89 mmHg) is associated with a 2.5- and 1.6-fold increase in cardiovascular (CV) disease in men and women respectively. A large proportion of cardiovascular disease is attributed to stage 1 (140–159/90–99 mmHg), which is the most prevalent among the stages of severity of hypertension.

7.5 **Systolic hypertension**

Risk of cardiovascular disease tends to increase progressively with systolic blood pressure. In the Framingham Heart Study, the incidence of coronary artery disease (CAD), stroke, and peripheral artery disease was higher for isolated systolic hypertension, mainly as result of arterial compliance. Isolated diastolic hypertension (HTn) which is more common in the young does not have any significant clinical impact. Treating elevated isolated systolic BP and a combination of both systolic and diastolic BP decreases the risk of cardiovascular disease.

7.6 **Left ventricular hypertrophy**

Hypertension is an important cause of left ventricular hypertrophy (LVH). Population studies have shown that it is an ominous harbinger of cardiovascular disease in the hypertensive patient. Risk of cardiovascular sequelae increases progressively with an increase in left ventricular mass and an increase in the severity of LVH by electrocardiography (ECG) criteria. A 39 g/m² increase in left ventricular mass/metre² confers a 40% increase in cardiovascular events. Hypertension plays a major role in the progression of heart failure. LVH is noted on the ECG in 20% of the heart failure cases and 60–70% is demonstrated by echocardiogram. Aggressive blood pressure control can prevent the development of LVH and reverse or regress it. Numerous clinical trials have shown the regression of LVH with blood pressure control. However, different group of drugs appear to cause regression of LVH to a different degree, as was seen in the Losartan Intervention for Endpoint (LIFE) reduction in Hypertension trial.

Studies, including reports from the Framingham Heart Study, suggest that regression of LVH confers an improvement in risk for cardiovascular disease. A substudy of the Heart Outcomes Prevention Evaluation (HOPE) trial examined whether treatment of high-risk patients with the angiotensin-converting inhibitor, ramipril, could prevent the development of LVH or promote its regression when compared with placebo in 8281 patients. The prevention or regression of LVH was noted in patients who were receiving active drug therapy whereas persistence or development of LVH was noted in patients who received placebo. Prevention or regression of LVH was associated with a 25% decrease in risk for cardiovascular disease. A decreased risk of developing heart failure was noted in patients who experienced prevention or regression of LVH.

LVH can also increase the risk of sudden death. This can be by mechanisms such as ventricular arrhythmias, heart failure, stroke, etc. LVH is discussed in more detail in Chapter 9.

7.7 **Conclusion**

Elevated blood pressure plays an important role in the determination of future cardiovascular morbidity and mortality. Antihypertensive therapy is associated with a 35–40%mean reduction in stroke incidence, 20–25% reduction myocardial infarction, and more than a 50% reduction in the incidence of heart failure. Treatment should be initiated after the confirmation of hypertension with a series of BP readings in the office. Physicians should provide every patient with their BP readings and their goals. Systolic blood pressure should be the focus of assessing risk and necessity of therapy. More often, hypertension is associated with metabolically driven risk factors like dyslipidemia, impaired glucose tolerance, hyperuricemia, and obesity, hence a thorough evaluation for these risk factors should be made at the time of treatment.

Key references

1988 Joint National Committee on detection, evaluation and treatment of high blood pressure (1988). The 1988 report of the Joint National Committee on detection, evaluation and treatment of high blood pressure. *Archives of Internal Medicine;* 148: 1023–38.

Belanger A, Cupples LA, D'Agostino RB (1988). *Means at each examination and inter-examination consistency of specified characteristics: Framingham Heart Study: 30-year follow-up.* US Dept of Health and Human Services, Washington DC. Public Health Service, National Institutes of Health document 80–2970.

Kannel WB, Dannenberg AJ, Levy D (1987). Population implications of electrocardiographic left ventricular hypertrophy. *American Journal of Cardiology;* 60: 851–931.

Kannel WB (1991). Epidemiology of essential hypertension: the Framingham experience. *Proceedings of the Royal College of Physicians Edinburgh;* 21: 273–87.

Levy D, Salomon M, D'Agostino RB, *et al.* (1994). Prognostic implications of baseline electrocardiographic features and their serial changes in subjects with left ventricular hypertrophy. *Circulation;* 90(4): 1786–93.

Lewington S, Clarke R, Qizilbash N, *et al.* (2002). Age-specific relevance of usual blood pressure to vascular mortality. *Lancet;* 360: 1903–13.

Mathew J, Sleight P, Lonn E, *et al.* for the Heart Outcomes Prevention Evaluation (HOPE) Investigators (2001). Reduction of cardiovascular risk by regression of electrocardiographic markers of left ventricular hypertrophy by the angiotensin-converting enzyme inhibitor ramipril. *Circulation;* 104: 1615–21.

Prospective studies collaboration, Lewington S, Whitlock G, Clarke R, *et al.* (2007). Blood cholesterol and vascular mortality by age, sex, and blood pressure: a meta-analysis of individual data from 61 prospective studies with 55,000 vascular deaths. *Lancet;* Dec 1; 370(9602): 1829–39.

Sundstrom J, Arima H, Jackson R, for the Blood pressure Lowering Treatment Trialists Collaboration (2014). Effects of blood pressure reduction in mild hypertension: A systematic review and meta analysis. *Annals of Internal Medicine;* December (Epub)

Turnbull F. (2003). Blood pressure lowering trialists collaboration (2003) Effects of different blood-pressure-lowering regimens on major cardiovascular events: results of prospectively-designed overviews of randomised trials *Lancet;* 8; 362(9395): 1527–35.

Vasan RS, Larson MG, Leip EP, *et al.* (2002). Residual life-time risk for developing hypertension in middle-aged women and men. The Framingham Heart Study. *Journal of American Medical Association;* Feb 27; 287(8): 1003–10.

Chapter 8

Target organ damage in hypertension

Sunil Nadar

Key points

- Hypertension is associated with a prothrombotic state.
- Platelet activation, endothelial dysfunction, and altered angiogenesis play an important part in the pathophysiology of target organ damage in hypertension.
- Target organ damage includes microvascular (retinopathy nephropathy, vascular dementia) and macrovascular injuries (stroke and myocardial infarctions).
- Good blood pressure control can help to delay the onset of this target organ damage.

8.1 Introduction

Hypertension is an important cardiovascular risk factor. As early as the 1970s, the significance of hypertension in the pathogenesis of atherothrombotic stroke was established, and newer studies continue to confirm the benefit achieved from blood pressure reduction in the prevention of cardiovascular and cerebrovascular diseases.

The high blood pressure that is associated with hypertension can also affect specific organ groups leading to the term 'target organ damage' (TOD), which in addition to the atherosclerotic vascular diseases mentioned above, include renal failure, retinopathy, vascular dementia, and left ventricular hypertrophy (LVH). Apart from blood pressure per se, many pathophysiological processes may contribute to the development of hypertensive TOD, as highlighted in Chapter 2.

For example, hypertension is associated with abnormalities in coagulation, platelets, and the endothelium, leading to a prothrombotic or hypercoagulable state. The latter may explain why despite the blood vessels being exposed to high pressures, the main complications of hypertension—that is, heart attacks and strokes—are thrombotic rather than haemorrhagic. In addition, there are other changes involving the renin–angiotensin–aldosterone system (RAAS), metalloproteinases, natriuretic peptides, etc., which could all influence the pathogenesis of the above mentioned TOD. LVH is a very important TOD and is discussed separately in the next chapter.

8.2 Hypertensive retinopathy

Hypertensive retinopathy is commonly seen in the eyes of patients with long-standing uncontrolled hypertension. These changes occur in the retina, optic nerve head, and choroidal circulation. The changes in the retina (hypertensive retinopathy) are the most widespread early changes that are seen and that have been described. There are many classifications for these changes, including the well-established Keith–Wagener–Barker classification and the Scheie classification. The Keith–Wagener–Barker classification was the first to try to correlate retinal findings with blood pressure (Table 8.1), whilst the Scheie classification (and the modified Scheie classification, see Box 8.1) was based on the fundoscopy findings alone. However, it is now thought that these classifications do not correlate well with the severity of hypertension and progression, and a new simpler two-grade classification of non-malignant versus malignant retinopathy has been proposed.

The most common ocular manifestation of hypertension is narrowing of the retinal arterioles. In young patients, the arterioles may constrict due to autoregulation as described in the following text. In older patients, luminal fibrosis and vessel rigidity prevent the same degree of narrowing. At points where the retinal arteriole crosses over the retinal venule, compression of the vein may cause the appearance of arteriovenous nicking. Other changes that are seen include cotton wool spots (nerve layer micro-infarcts that obtain this appearance due to disruption of axoplasmic transport), dot/blot hemorrhages, and flame-shaped haemorrhages (Figure 8.1).

Under normal circumstances, there are many feedback mechanisms that maintain retinal flow despite changes in blood pressure. Retinal vessels have the ability to maintain a constant blood flow despite changes in perfusion pressures by either vasodilation or vasoconstriction. However, with hypertension, there is a breakdown of this mechanism, due to changes in endothelial-derived molecules (endothelins, thromboxane A2, etc.). This breakdown of the autoregulation leads to other changes such as oedema and fibrosis. In malignant hypertension, the changes seen include papilloedema as well as hard and soft exudates which are due to severe vasospasm of the vessels in response to the high pressures (as seen in malignant hypertension), leading to necrosis and focal leakage from the precapillary arterioles that lie deep in the retina.

Table 8.1 The Keith–Wagener–Barker classification

	Fundoscopy findings	Clinical correlates
Grade 1	Slight narrowing, sclerosis, and tortuosity of the retinal arterioles	Mild asymptomatic hypertension
Grade 2	Definite narrowing, focal constriction, sclerosis, and arteriovenous (AV) nicking	Blood pressure is higher and sustained, few if any symptoms attributable to high blood pressure
Grade 3	Cotton wool spots, haemorrhages	Blood pressure higher and more sustained, symptoms such as headaches, vertigo
Grade 4	As above, with papilloedema, Elschnig spots	Persistently elevated blood pressure, headaches, visual disturbances, impaired cerebral and renal function

Box 8.1 Modified Scheie classification of hypertensive retinopathy

Grade 0 No changes
Grade 1 Minimal arteriolar narrowing
Grade 2 Obvious arteriolar narrowing with focal irregularities
Grade 3 Grade 2 + retinal hemorrhages and/or exudate
Grade 4 Grade 3 + swollen optic nerve (malignant hypertension)

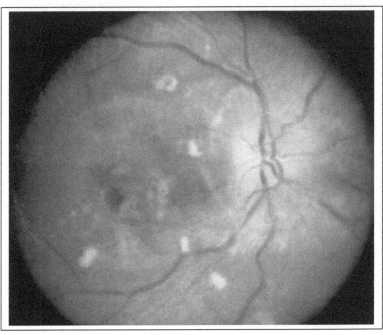

Figure 8.1 Fundoscopy showing malignant hypertensive changes with papilloedema, haemorrhages, infarcts (cotton wool spots), and arteriolar constriction

8.3 **Cognitive impairment/vascular dementia**

The inverse association between blood pressure and cognitive impairment has been demonstrated in a number of epidemiological and treatment studies. The Framingham Heart Study was one of the first to demonstrate that attention and memory measures are inversely related to blood pressure levels and duration of hypertension. This was later proved in other large epidemiological studies.

What mechanisms involved here are not certain. Hypertension is a risk factor for atherosclerosis, stroke, or cerebral infarction, which in turn may cause cognitive decline. In the absence of an overt cerebrovascular accident or stroke, cognitive impairment may be a result of occlusion of microvasculature. Patients with hypertension have smaller volumes of thalamic nuclei and larger volumes of cerebrospinal fluid in the cerebellum and temporal lobes.

The Systolic hypertension in Europe Study (Syst Eur) was one of the first studies to demonstrate a protective effect of antihypertensive therapy on the development of cognitive impairment. Similar findings have been demonstrated in larger studies including the Perindopril Protection Against Recurrent Stroke Study (PROGRESS) and the Study on Cognition and Prognosis in the Elderly (SCOPE). Antihypertensive therapy has also been shown to reduce the incidence of white matter changes on magnetic resonance imaging.

8.4 Hypertensive renal disease

Renal disease has an important relationship with hypertension in that it could be either be a cause or an effect of hypertension. It is epidemiologically more common to see renal failure leading to hypertension, but the converse is controversial, except in malignant hypertension, where progressive deterioration of renal function has been demonstrated.

The mechanisms involved here are similar to those seen for the retinal disease. Here as well, the glomerular vessels autoregulate the blood flow by vasoconstriction or vasodilatation depending on the perfusion pressures, to keep the actual perfusion at the glomerulus constant. Prolonged high perfusion pressures can lead to significant vasoconstriction, which can then cause localized damage to the glomeruli. This can cause necrosis of the glomeruli leading to microalbuminuria, which could lead to significant proteinuria if the disease is not treated. Renal failure in the absence of the malignant phase could also be an effect of atherosclerosis affecting the renal arteries, leading to underperfusion.

As with LVH, microalbuminuria has also been shown to correlate with future cardiovascular events. The reversal of microalbuminuria with the strict treatment of hypertension has been shown to improve cardiovascular events.

8.5 Molecular mechanisms involved

As seen earlier, hypertension can cause changes in many organ systems. There are many factors involved and no factor, on its own, can be singled out as the most important one. It is an interaction of these various factors that causes the effects noted in the various organ systems.

8.5.1 Changes in the endothelium

The changes in the endothelium in hypertension are widespread and well established. This activated endothelium causes increased production of procoagulant and inflammatory agents and is associated with a shift of the actions of the endothelium towards reduced vasodilation, a pro-inflammatory state, and prothrombic properties. With constant exposure to this high-pressure flow, and as a result of the inflammatory mediators and the effects of the neutrophils and platelets that have got adhered to the endothelium, it then starts to become dysfunctional. This 'dysfunctional' or 'damaged' or 'activated' endothelium then sets up a vicious cycle whereby the blood pressure tends to remain elevated due to changes in the NO and endothelin bioavailability.

This activated endothelium sets up a chain of events that include decreased NO activity, elevated endothelins, elevated levels of tissue plasminogen activator (tPA) and plasminogen activator inhibitor (PAI), and an increase in the levels of angiotensin-converting enzyme (ACE).

Endothelial dysfunction is associated with different cardiovascular risk factors such as ageing, postmenopausal status, hypercholesterolemia, diabetes mellitus, smoking, hyperhomocysteinaemia, and hypertension. It is also detectable in the presence of coronary atherosclerosis. Combination of these risk factors has been shown to lead to further deterioration of the endothelial-dependent vasodilatation.

This is especially important as changes in NO also have effects on platelet aggregation, smooth muscle proliferation, and migration, as well as monocyte adhesion and adhesion molecule expression that play an important role in the genesis of thrombosis and atherosclerotic plaque. Therefore, endothelial dysfunction is now considered a relevant mechanism that promotes atherosclerosis and thrombosis.

Recently, it has been shown that levels of endothelial damage in hypertensive patients are related to the presence or absence of TOD as well as to cardiovascular risk and prognosis. Conceivably, endothelial function can also be used as an intermediary end point in the treatment of hypertension.

8.5.2 **Platelets**

Platelets from patients with hypertension differ morphologically and biochemically from those in normotensive subjects and it is well accepted that platelets from patients with hypertension are in a state of activation. Platelets get activated in hypertension for a variety of reasons. These include the increased shear force that platelets are exposed to, neuroendocrine factors, such as increase in angiotensin II levels and catecholamines, and endothelial dysfunction.

It should be noted that other comorbidities, such as atrial fibrillation, diabetes, and congestive heart failure are more common in hypertensive patients, and are known to activate platelets. Conceivably, some consider that the atherosclerotic lesions that are seen with hypertensive patients could act as a nidus for further platelet activation.

8.5.3 **Thrombogenesis**

Hypertension is associated with a prothrombotic state. Although the condition is associated with high pressures, it is commonly complicated by thrombotic events such as ischaemic strokes and myocardial infarctions. This is the thrombotic paradox of hypertension. This is because hypertension fulfils the criteria of Virchow's triad for thrombosis. There is alteration in blood flow due to the increased shear forces. There is vessel wall change with changes to the endothelium. Platelet activation fulfills the third criterion of alteration to the blood constituents.

Many changes in the coagulation and fibrinolytic pathways of hypertensive patients have been documented. These changes suggest increase in coagulability and impaired fibrinolysis. For example, activity of tPA and levels of PAI antigen have been shown to be higher in hypertensives than in non-hypertensive patients. Fibrin D-dimer, an index of fibrin turnover and thrombogenesis, has also been shown to be raised in hypertensives. Plasma fibrin D-dimer levels are predictive of both arterial thrombotic events and postoperative thrombosis.

8.5.4 **Changes in matrix metalloproteinases**

The matrix metalloproteinases (MMPs) are a family of zinc-dependent endoproteinases with the combined ability to degrade all the components of extracellular matrix at a physiological pH. Tissue inhibitors of these MMPs (TIMPs) have also been described and they tend to keep the action of MMPs under check. Imbalances between the levels of TIMPs and MMPs could therefore lead to changes in the extracellular matrix. In hypertension, it has been shown that there is a decrease in the levels of the collagenases and an increase in the levels of their inhibitors, leading to an increase in the laying down of the extracellular matrix.

Correlations of levels of MMP and TIMPs have also been demonstrated in hypertensives with the presence or absence of microalbuminuria and a prothrombotic state. Recent clinical studies have shown that the levels of MMPs are altered in hypertension and that these correlate with cardiovascular risk and the presence of LVH and improve with treatment of hypertension.

8.5.5 **Changes in angiotensin II**

The RAAS plays a very important role in the maintenance of a normal blood pressure. The endothelial dysfunction that occurs in hypertension can lead to alterations in the RAAS. In hypertension that is related to a high angiotensin II or high renin state, increased levels of angiotensin II could contribute to the increased vascular thickness and stiffness that is seen in hypertensives. This is especially important, as it has been shown that high plasma renin activity in hypertensive patients is associated with increased risk for coronary events and stroke.

8.5.6 **Altered angiogenesis**

Altered angiogenesis in hypertension has been well documented. The microcirculation is important in regulation of peripheral vascular tone and it is altered in hypertension. It has been demonstrated that in essential hypertension, there is small vessel rarefaction and an absence of angiogenesis. The exact mechanism of this is not known. However, it has been suggested that vessel wall thickening and a response of the muscular wall of the vessels to increased flow and blood pressures causes this rarefaction. This vasoconstriction of the peripheral vessels causes increased peripheral resistance, which then perpetuates the increased blood pressure and sets up a vicious cycle. Endothelial dysfunction, as discussed earlier, also occurs with decrease in NO, leading to further peripheral vasoconstriction. Pulse pressure, mean arterial pressure, and pressure wave, along with cardiac output, also affect microcirculation.

Recent studies have shown increase in plasma levels of vascular endothelial growth factor (VEGF) and angiopoietins in hypertensives. These levels correlate well with cardiovascular risk and improve with treatment. It has been suggested that increase in angiogenic factors is a compensatory mechanism as a result of tissue hypoxia due to the rarefaction of the microcirculation.

8.6 **Summary**

As seen earlier, many pathogenetic mechanisms are at work in hypertension. Most of these changes are interrelated (Figure 8.2). The endothelial dysfunction and platelet activation lead to changes including increase in angiotensin II levels, which in turn leads to smooth muscle proliferation and collagen deposition by altering levels of matrix metalloproteins. These changes are responsible for the microvascular disease such as retinopathy and nephropathy and could

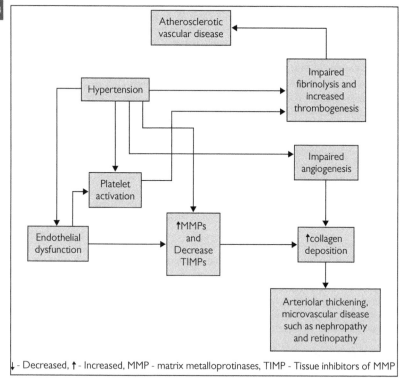

↓ - Decreased, ↑ - Increased, MMP - matrix metalloprotinases, TIMP - Tissue inhibitors of MMP

Figure 8.2 The interactions between the different factors in the pathogenesis of target organ damage

also influence LVH. The increase in thrombogenesis, impaired fibrinolysis, and platelet activation could be responsible for macrovascular diseases such as strokes and peripheral vascular disease, whilst all the changes together could result in increased atherogenesis.

The main aim in the management of a patient with hypertension is the prevention of cardiovascular and cerebrovascular complications. The importance of good blood pressure control towards this end cannot be overemphasized. Medical literature is full of studies demonstrating the clinical benefits of good blood pressure control in preventing cardiovascular and cerebrovascular endpoints, irrespective of the agent used. Recent studies also show that it is the ambulatory blood pressure control over 24 hours that gives a better indication of the patient's risk of cardiovascular endpoints rather than the office blood pressure readings.

An understanding of the different pathophysiological mechanisms involved in the causation of TOD in hypertension is important, as this would help us devise means of reducing catastrophic complications of hypertension. Whilst it has been shown convincingly that the use of antihypertensive agents reduces cardiovascular and cerebrovascular complications and that they reverse endothelial and platelet activation in hypertension, a direct correlation between the improvement in endothelial and platelet activation and a decrease in cardiovascular endpoints has not been shown. More studies are needed to fully understand the different mechanisms involved in the pathogenesis of target organ damage in hypertension and in devising strategies to prevent them.

Key references

Cuspidi C, Rescaldani M, Tadic M, et al. (2015). White coate hypertension as defined by ambulatory blood pressure monitoring and subclinical cardiac organ damage: a meta-analysis. *Journal of Hypertension*; 33:24–32.

Forette F, Seux ML, Staessen JA, et al. (2002). The prevention of dementia with antihypertensive treatment: new evidence from the Systolic Hypertension in Europe (Syst-Eur) study. *Archives of Internal Medicine*; 162: 2046–52.

Kaplan NM (1998). The endothelium as prognostic factor and therapeutic target: what criteria should we apply? *Journal of Cardiovascular Pharmacology*; 32(Suppl 3): S78–S80.

Lithell H, Hansson L, Skoog I, et al. (2003). The Study on Cognition and Prognosis in the Elderly (SCOPE): principal results of a randomized double-blind intervention trial. *Journal of Hypertension*; 21: 875–86.

Mayet J, Hughes A (2003). Cardiac and vascular pathophysiology in hypertension. *Heart*; 89: 1104–9.

Muiesan M, Salvetti M, Rizzoni D (2013) Resistant hypertension and target organ damage. *Hypertension Research*; 36:485–91

Nadar S, Lip GY (2003). The prothrombotic state in hypertension and the effects of antihypertensive treatment. *Current Pharmaceutical Design*; 9(21): 1715–32.

Nadar S, Blann AD, Lip GY (2004). Endothelial dysfunction: methods of assessment and application to hypertension. *Current Pharmaceutical Design*; 10(29): 3591–605.

Nadar SK, Tayebjee MH, Messerli F, et al. (2006). Target organ damage in hypertension: pathophysiology and implications for drug therapy. *Current Pharmaceutical Design*; 12(13): 1581–92.

Ong YT, Wong TY, Klein R, et al. (2013). Hypertensive retinopathy and the risk of stroke *Hypertension*; 62:706–11.

Perticone F, Ceravolo R, Pujia A, et al. (2001). Prognostic significance of endothelial dysfunction in hypertensive patients. *Circulation*; 104: 191–6.

Schwartz GL, Strong CG (1987). Renal parenchymal involvement in essential hypertension. *Medicine Clinics of North America*; 71: 843–58.

Tzourio C, Anderson C (2000). Blood pressure reduction and risk of dementia in patients with stroke: rationale of the dementia assessment in PROGRESS (Perindopril Protection Against Recurrent Stroke Study). PROGRESS Management Committee. *Journal of Hypertension Supplement*; 18: S21–S24.

Chapter 9

Left ventricular hypertrophy

Sunil Nadar

Key points

- Left ventricular hypertrophy (LVH) is a well-known complication of long-standing hypertension, with the duration and severity of the elevated blood pressure being the major predictive factors in its development.

- The renin–angiotensin–aldosterone system (RAAS) has been implicated as the main pathophysiological mechanism in its development.

- The presence of LVH in hypertensive patients is a poor prognostic factor and those with LVH are at a higher cardiovascular risk for future events.

- The regression of LVH with the treatment of hypertension can lead to a corresponding reduction in cardiovascular risk.

- Antihypertensive agents acting on the RAAS appear to be best at regressing LVH and in improving outcomes.

9.1 Introduction

Left ventricular hypertrophy (LVH) is a common finding in hypertensives and is an important manifestation of hypertensive target organ damage (TOD) in them. A recent meta-analysis suggests that the prevalence of LVH varies from 36–41% of a pooled population of hypertensive patients. Its prevalence is similar in males and females. LVH is predominantly related to the duration of hypertension and the levels of elevated blood pressures. The pathophysiological mechanisms involved in LVH include a general hypertrophy of the muscles in response to contracting against a high arterial pressure. In the initial stages, LVH is therefore a compensatory process that represents an adaptation to increased ventricular wall stress.

Systolic and diastolic pressures are both closely related to LV mass and wall thickness respectively, suggesting an influence of both volume and pressure load on hypertension-related LVH. Overall, the presence of LVH substantially increases the risk of stroke, coronary heart disease, congestive heart failure, and arrhythmias.

9.2 Diagnosis of LVH

The diagnosis of LVH is made by both electrocardiography (ECG) and echocardiogram examination. Table 9.1 lists the common criteria that are used for the diagnosis of LVH. As ECG is often the first test that is done in patients with hypertension, there is a need for good diagnostic criteria. However, none of these criteria are universally accepted as evidenced by different clinical trials using different criteria for the diagnosis of LVH. None of the criteria that are currently used have a good sensitivity; however, they are fairly specific.

Table 9.1 ECG criteria for diagnosing LVH			
	Criteria	Sensitivity (%)	Specificity (%)
Cornell criteria	RaVL plus an S wave in V3 greater than 2.8 mV in men or greater than 2.0 mV in women	22	95
Cornell voltage-duration	Cornell voltage × QRS duration	95	50–60
Sokolow–Lyon criteria	S wave in V1 plus an R wave in V5 or V6 greater than 3.5 mV or an R wave in V5 or V6 greater than 2.6 mV	25	95
Gubner-Ungerleider criteria	R wave in I plus an S wave in III greater than 2.5 mV	13	95
Romhilt-Estes scoring system	Excessive amplitude: 3 points (largest R or S wave in limb leads ≥ 20 mV or S wave in V1 or V2 ≥ 30 mV or R wave in V5 or V6 ≥ 30 mV). ST-T segment pattern of LV strain: 3 points (ST-T segment vector shifted in direction opposite to mean QRS vector). Left atrial involvement: 3 points (terminal negativity of P wave in V1 ≥ 1 mm with duration ≥ 0.04 s). Left axis deviation: 2 points (left axis ≥ −30° in frontal plain). Prolonged QRS duration: 1 point (≥ 0.09 s). Intrinsicoid deflection: 1 point (intrinsicoid deflection in V5 or V6 ≥ 0.05 s). Two thresholds in use: positive if ≥ 4 points or ≥ 5 points	50	95

Echocardiogram continues to be the gold standard for the diagnosis of LVH, although other modalities of imaging such as magnetic resonance imaging or CT scanning may also be helpful in making the diagnosis.

LVH is diagnosed based on the calculation of the LV mass. LV mass is derived from the formula described by Devereux and colleagues. Thus, the LV mass (in grams) is calculated as $0.8 \times 1.04 [(IVSd + LVIDd + LVPWd)^3 - (LVID)^3] + 0.6$, where IVSd is the interventricular septal thickness in diastole, LVIDd is the left ventricular internal diameter in diastole, and LVPDd is the left ventricular posterior wall at end diastole. Other indices used are the relative wall thickness (RWT), (the ratio of twice the LVPWd and the LVID) and the LV mass index (LVMI) which is calculated as the LV mass corrected for body surface area. LVMI is a more accurate measure of LVH than just LV mass as it takes into account the patient's age, sex, race, and body habitus, all of which can influence LV mass.

As left ventricular (LV) mass is a continuous variable, the threshold value for LVH is arbitrary; however, LVH is often defined as the upper 5% of the distribution of LV mass in the population. There is no clear consensus concerning the cut-off values used to define LVH with echo. An LVMI of 131 g/m² for men and 100 g/m² for women derived from echo measurements was used to define the lower limit of LVH in the Framingham study whereas the corresponding figures were 117 g/m² and 104 g/m² in a study by De Simone and 125 g/m² and 110 g/m² in the 2003 ESC guidelines.

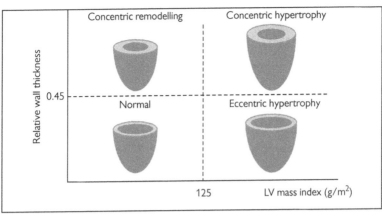

Figure 9.1 The four types of LV geometry

9.3 **Pathophysiology and development of LVH**

There are four distinct patterns of LV geometry in hypertension (Figure 9.1). Normal LV geometry is identified by normal LV mass and a normal relation between the cavity size and the wall thickness such as RWT. Concentric remodelling is characterized by a normal LV mass but an increased RWT (RWT > 0.45). Eccentric LVH is characterized by a large LV size but a normal RWT (RWT < 0.45); it is related to volume load and may be a physiologic adaptation to dynamic exercise and is also common in obesity. Morphologically, eccentric LVH shows a relative increase in the number of myocytes. Concentric LVH occurs in conditions associated with pressure overload and is related to static exercise. LVH is a pathological condition with a relative increase in connective tissue and fibrosis often found in hypertension. In a pooled meta-analysis population, eccentric LVH was found to be the most common type of hypertrophy followed by concentric LVH.

Arterial pressure is the predominant haemodynamic factor and is usually the most powerful determinant of LV mass in hypertensive patients. However, the relatively low correlation coefficients between blood pressure and LV mass suggests that there are other mechanisms and factors that are equally, if not more, important. Other demographic determinants such as age, race, sex, and body size are all known to play a role in the development of LV mass.

Non-haemodynamic risk factors of the development of LVH include trophic factors mediated by the sympathetic nervous system, the renin–angiotensin–aldosterone system (RAAS) and insulin. Activation of the sympathetic nervous system has long been implicated in the development of LVH. Although *in vitro* studies appear to show a correlation between the two, *in vivo* studies have not been that definite. It also appears that LVH is related to the haemodynamic changes elicited by sympathetic nerve activation rather than to a direct adrenergic effect on the myocardium.

Patients with LVH often have increased levels of insulin and insulin resistance. Insulin has trophic effects, and insulin resistance is more common among hypertensive patients than in normotensive subjects. Insulin resistance is associated with an attenuated therapeutic response to antihypertensive drugs. In contrast, the role of the RAAS in the development of LVH is much clearer. Circulating plasma levels of aldosterone and angiotensin II are related to the extent of LVH. It has been suggested that angiotensin II promotes myocyte cell growth and aldosterone may increase the collagen content and stimulate the development of myocardial fibrosis. Circumstantial evidence in support of an important role for the RAAS in the causation of LVH is provided by the effects of treatments aimed at blocking the RAAS and will be discussed later in the chapter.

Leptin, a 16kDa protein hormone that plays a key role in regulating energy intake and expenditure, has recently been found to be associated with LV growth. Fasting plasma leptin levels strongly correlate with echocardiographic determinants of LVH. In newly diagnosed hypertensives, fasting plasma leptin levels determine myocardial wall thickness independently of 24-hour ambulatory blood pressure levels.

A study on the 24-hour blood pressure patterns in 35 non-diabetic renal transplant recipients with the presence or absence of LVH demonstrated that the absence of a nocturnal fall in blood pressure (non-dipper status) is associated with a higher incidence of LVH. In addition, another study found that pulse pressure most significantly predicted the incidence of LVH on follow-up. This is important as pulse pressure does reflect the elasticity of the blood vessels, and perhaps suggests that the same mechanisms that cause vessel inelasticity and thickening are responsible for LVH.

The role of dietary salt in the pathogenesis of LVH was first described by Schmeider in 1988. Since then others have also confirmed this to be true. It has been suggested that increased sodium intake increases the preload and thereby increases LVH. It has also been suggested to work via the RAAS and via the sympathetic nervous system. The different aetiological factors have been summarized in Figure 9.2.

LVH can also occur in trained athletes and is considered to be a normal adaptation, commonly called physiologic LVH. This differentiation is important as physiological LVH is reversible, and does not seem to be associated with adverse prognosis as is pathological LVH secondary to hypertension. Although it is difficult to distinguish the two forms of LVH by electrocardiogram or echocardiography, some reports suggest that physiological LVH demonstrates normal diastolic filling patterns whilst pathological LVH shows signs of diastolic dysfunction.

9.4 **Prognostic aspects of hypertensive LVH**

Casale and colleagues (1986) were among the first to demonstrate the relationship between adverse outcomes in hypertensive patients with LVH in a follow-up study of 140 men with uncomplicated hypertension over five years. Subsequent studies including the Framingham Heart Study have since shown a direct relationship between LVH at baseline examination and the risk of subsequent morbid or mortal events in clinical or epidemiological populations.

Indeed, subjects with LVH have a two- to fourfold higher rate of cardiovascular complications independent of other risk factors such as hypercholesterolemia, age, and blood pressure measured in the clinic. This relationship is independent of other factors such as age, gender, blood pressure, smoking, cholesterol, and diabetes. Table 9.2 summarizes some of the major studies on prognosis and LVH.

LVH also predicts the development of stroke and atrial fibrillation. In the Framingham cohort, echocardiographic LVH was found to be predictive of incident stroke. After adjusting for other risk factors, the hazard ratio (HR) for stroke and transient ischaemic attack was 1.5 (95% confidence interval [CI],1.2–1.8) for each quartile increment in height-adjusted LV mass. This relationship has also been demonstrated in a cohort of African Americans in the Atheroscleoris in the Communities (ARIC) study.

The development of atrial fibrillation in patients with LVH may be one pathway by which LVH can lead to strokes. For example, it has been shown that for every 1 standard deviation increase in LV mass, the risk of atrial fibrillation was increased by 1.2-fold.

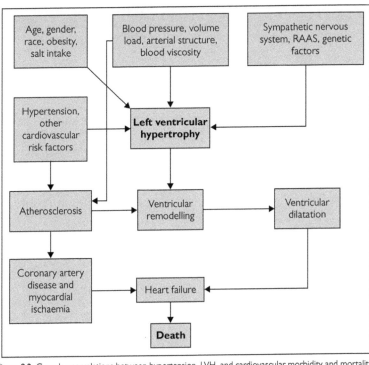

Figure 9.2 Complex correlations between hypertension, LVH, and cardiovascular morbidity and mortality

LVH has also been associated with sudden cardiac death. Patients with LVH have an increased risk for ventricular arrhythmias after adjusting for other risk factors for ventricular ectopy. The predisposition to ventricular arrhythmias in LVH may be related to action potential prolongation, increased dispersion of refractoriness, and lowering of the ventricular fibrillation threshold.

Several mechanisms have been proposed to explain the increased cardiovascular risk associated with LVH. The most commonly proposed factor is that LVH serves as a surrogate marker for other risk factors. LVH is a measure of preclinical cardiac disease and is closely related to systemic atherosclerosis. It correlates with carotid artery diameter and carotid intimal medial thickness. LVH is also associated with diastolic dysfunction as a result of myocardial fibrosis. This fibrosis may be mediated by angiotensin II.

The pattern of hypertrophy also plays some role in the adverse prognosis related to LVH. Concentric hypertrophy appears to carry the highest risk and eccentric hypertrophy an intermediate risk. The reason for this difference in prognosis for the different geometric patterns is not certain. The eccentric pattern of LV mass distribution is considered to reflect normal mass to volume distribution, whilst the concentric pattern is more suggestive of a response to volume or pressure overload. This pattern is associated with severe haemodynamic and structural abnormalities and would therefore represent a more unfavorable pattern.

Table 9.2 Studies demonstrating cardiovascular benefit with LVH regression		
Authors, country, year	Subjects and methods	Findings
Muiesan, Italy, 1995	215 hypertensive patients (men and women) followed up for ten years	Cardiovascular events were more in those without regression of LVH. In those with regression, the event rates were similar to those without baseline LVH
Verdecchia, Italy, 1998	430 hypertensive patients (men and women) followed up for seven to ten years	Event rate was 1.58 per 100 person years among those who achieved regression versus 6.27 for those who did not achieve LVH regression
Cipriano, France, 2001	474 hypertensive patients followed up for five years	Incidence of cardiovascular events was 4.8% in the group without LVH both before and during treatment, 9.6% in the group with LVH regression and 15% in the group without regression of LVH
Koren, USA, 2002	172 patients followed up for five years	Event rate in those with LVH regression was 8.8% while it was 19.8% in those without LVH regression

LVH can also lead to increased mortality and morbidity by other mechanisms including an increased risk of arrhythmias, diastolic dysfunction, decreased contractility, and impaired coronary reserve.

9.5 **Treatment and regression of LVH**

It has been long noticed that treatment of hypertension can lead to regression of LVH. Almost six decades ago it was first demonstrated that cardiac hypertrophy could be reversed by nephrectomy in spontaneously hypertensive rats. At around the same time, similar results were demonstrated in human hypertensive patients as well, initially with the regression of ECG features of LVH following treatment of blood pressures. However, the prognostic benefits related to regression of LVH above and beyond the benefits related to the changes in blood pressure and other risk factors have not been fully appreciated until recently. In general, few studies are powered sufficiently to detect the prognostic impact of serial changes of LVH either at ECG or echocardiography in hypertensive subjects.

In the Framingham Heart Study, the subjects with baseline LVH who showed an increase over time in the ECG voltages were twice as likely to suffer a cardiovascular event over the subsequent years as compared with those with a decrease in the voltages. A substudy of the Heart Outcomes Prevention Evaluation (HOPE) study (which compared the effects of ramipril in addition to standard therapy, with placebo and vitamin E in about 9500 patients at high risk for cardiovascular events) demonstrated that the rate of strokes, heart attacks, and cardiovascular deaths among those who did not develop LVH or experienced regression was 12.3%, while the rate was 15.8% among individuals who developed LVH or experienced no regression.

The risk of developing congestive heart failure was 9.3% among those with regression or prevention and 15.4% in the group with LVH development or persistence.

Subsequently, there have been many studies that showed that regression of LVH with treatment appears to decrease the chance of cardiovascular morbidity and mortality, and improved left ventricular diastolic function (Table 9.2). A recent substudy of the LIFE study has also demonstrated that regression of LVH was associated with fewer admissions for heart failure.

Different antihypertensives appear to have different effects on LVH regression, as has indeed been demonstrated by the Losartan Intervention For Endpoint reduction (LIFE) study and in a meta-analysis by Klingbeil and colleagues. This meta-analysis studied more than 80 trials with 146 active treatment arms ($n = 3767$ patients) and 17 placebo arms ($n = 346$ patients). After adjusting for various variables, there was a significant difference among the different medication classes. The use of angiotensin II receptor blockers (ARBs) decreased LVMI by 13%. There was a reduction in LVMI by 11% with calcium antagonists, 10% with angiotensin-converting enzyme (ACE) inhibitors, and 8% with diuretics, and 6% with beta blockers. In pairwise comparisons, ARBs, calcium antagonists, and ACE inhibitors were more effective at reducing LV mass than were beta blockers.

Similar results have been obtained by the PRESERVE (Prospective Randomized Enalapril Study Evaluating Regression of Ventricular Enlargement) study, and the LIVE (LVH regression Indapamide Enalapril) study. In the latter study, indapamide caused similar regression of LVH as compared to enalapril. The meta-analysis mentioned earlier also found that direct vasodilators (such as hydralazine and minoxidil) may not cause LVH regression despite their blood pressure control. This could be due to reflex stimulation of the RAAS, sympathetic nervous system, and other trophic hormone release by these vasodilators, which may directly promote the development of LVH. Clonidine and prazosin may also be ineffective in causing LVH regression.

Recently aldosterone blockade with spironolactone has also been shown to cause LVH regression. Similar findings were also noted with eplerenone, which caused similar reductions in LV mass as compared to enalapril, but significantly higher reductions when the two drugs were combined.

Endothelin receptors are a new group of agents that are being trialled in humans. Endothelin is known to be a potent vasoconstrictor that is implicated in the pathogenesis of hypertension. It promotes the growth of myocytes and collagen synthesis by cardiac fibroblasts resulting in LVH. However, clinical trial data on their effect on reversing LVH are still awaited but preliminary data are encouraging.

9.6 How does LVH regression translate into clinical outcomes?

The mechanisms by which changes in LVH translate into clinical outcomes are not clear, but several theories have been proposed. There is evidence that several factors may induce simultaneous changes in LV mass and the atherosclerotic burden. As mentioned earlier, in hypertensive patients, LV mass and carotid intimal medial thickness correlate strongly. Therefore, with treatment, LVH regression could just be a surrogate marker for regression of atherosclerotic plaques.

Also important is the role of the RAAS. Angiotensin II and angiotensin II type 1 receptor activation promote intracellular reactions that include proliferation of vascular smooth muscle cells and production of extracellular matrix protein. These in turn lead to LVH and increase in atherosclerosis. The fact that ARBs were the most potent at reducing LVH lends credence to the theory that the RAAS is of great importance in the production and regression of LVH.

Regression of LVH may be achieved through a reduction in myocyte volume and amount of interstitium. Studies of regression of severe LVH in patients undergoing aortic valve replacement showed an initial and rapid reduction in the myocyte volume, followed by a more prolonged phase of progressive reduction in the interstitial fibrosis. This has been demonstrated in a study in hypertensive humans which included serial myocardial biopsies during the treatment with lisinopril. There have also been studies demonstrating regression of LVH with salt restriction. Furthermore, a low-salt diet also appears to improve the LVH regression that is caused by antihypertensive agents.

9.7 Implications for hypertension management

As discussed earlier, the data would suggest that regression of LVH should be a target in the treatment of hypertension. With the exception of minoxidil and hydralazine, most classes of hypertensive drugs have been shown to cause some regression of LVH. The data that are available at present suggest that inhibition of the RAAS and possibly calcium-channel blockade achieve the greatest reduction in LV mass. These effects appear to be independent of their blood pressure–lowering effect.

Regression of LVH in treated hypertensive subjects should thus be considered as a favourable prognostic marker that reflects a reduced risk of subsequent cardiovascular disease. In contrast, the patients with persistence or lack of regression of LVH over time should be considered at elevated cardiovascular risk even in the presence of a normal achieved blood pressure. An aggressive therapeutic management directed at achieving a blood pressure reduction over a 24-hour period and a strict control of concomitant modifiable risk factors seem mandatory in these high-risk patients.

Key references

Benjamin EJ, Levy D (1999). Why is left ventricular hypertrophy so predictive of morbidity and mortality? *American Journal of the Medical Sciences*; 317(3): 168–75.

Cuspidi C, Sala C, Negri F, et al (2012). Prevalence of left-ventricular hypertrophy in hypertension: an updated review of echocardiographic studies. *Journal of Human Hypertension*; 26(6): 343–49

Devereux RB, Alonso DR, Lutas EM, et al. (1986). Echocardiographic assessment of left ventricular hypertrophy: comparison to necropsy findings. *American Journal of Cardiology*; 57(6): 450–58.

Kahan T (1998). The importance of left ventricular hypertrophy in human hypertension. *Journal of Hypertension Supplement*; 16(7): S23–S29.

Klingbeil AU, Schneider M, Martus P, et al. (2003). A meta-analysis of the effects of treatment on left ventricular mass in essential hypertension. *American Journal of Medicine*; 115(1): 41–6.

Levy D (1988). Left ventricular hypertrophy. Epidemiological insights from the Framingham Heart Study. *Drugs*; 35(Suppl 5): 1–5.

Levy D, Savage DD, Garrison RJ, et al. (1987). Echocardiographic criteria for left ventricular hypertrophy: the Framingham Heart Study. *American Journal of Cardiology*; 59: 956–60.

Okin PM, Wachtell K, Gerdts E, et al. (2014). Relationship between left ventricular systolic function to persistence or development of electrocardiographic left ventricular hypertrophy in hypertensive patients: implications for the development of new heart failure. *Journal of Hypertension*; 32:2472–78.

Pewsner D, Jüni P, Egger M, et al. (2007). Accuracy of electrocardiography in diagnosis of left ventricular hypertrophy in arterial hypertension: systematic review. *British Medical Journal*; 335(7622): 711.

Schmieder RE, Martus P, Klingbeil A (1996). Reversal of left ventricular hypertrophy in essential hypertension. A meta-analysis of randomized double-blind studies. *Journal of American Medical Association*; 275(19): 1507–13.

Urhausen A, Kindermann W (1999). Sports-specific adaptations and differentiation of the athlete's heart. *Sports Medicine*; 28(4): 237–44.

Chapter 10

Atrial fibrillation and hypertension

Kully Sandhu and Shamil Yusuf

> **Key points**
>
> - Hypertension is considered to be an important risk factor for the development of atrial fibrillation.
> - Left atrial changes in hypertension are thought to be responsible for the development of atrial fibrillation.
> - Angiotensin-converting enzyme and angiotensin receptor blockers appear to delay the development of atrial fibrillation in hypertensives.

10.1 Introduction

Atrial fibrillation (AF) is well recognized to be the most prevalent clinically significant arrhythmia affecting 1–2% of the population. There are currently over 6 million Europeans experiencing AF and this is expected to double within the next 50 years. An insurance claims database that represented a diverse 5% of U.S population from 2001–2008 extrapolated that AF incidence will double from 1.2 million patients in 2010 to 2.6 million in 2030. This relates to the prevalence of 5.2 million in 2010 to 12.1 million patients in 2030.

Hypertension is the most prevalent cardiovascular disorder affecting 20–50% of the adult population in developed nations with increasing prevalence in developing nations. Both hypertension and AF are associated with increasing age. Therefore it comes as no surprise that hypertension is the most prevalent concomitant condition in patients with atrial fibrillation in Europe and North America and they are thought to be inextricably linked. There are a number of well-recognized risk factors for the predisposition of AF (Box 10.1); however, hypertension due to its prevalence remains the main risk factor, doubling the risk of AF. Interestingly, 'high normal' blood pressure has been linked with the development of atrial fibrillation. This is of great importance as high normal hypertension is potentially a reversible causative factor

AF is associated with increased overall mortality due to its association with stroke, heart failure, and recurrent hospitalizations. Therefore the importance of reversing or prevention of new atrial fibrillation should not be underestimated. Patients with atrial fibrillation have a 40–90% higher risk of overall mortality when compared to patients in sinus rhythm. Two of the most important cardiovascular complications associated with AF are cardiac failure and a four- to fivefold increase in thrombo-embolic stroke. Moreover, there is a threefold increase in stroke among patients with both AF and hypertension when compared with patients with AF alone. Furthermore a reduction of cardiac output by as much as 15–20% has been observed in patients induced with AF by right ventricular pacing.

Studies investigating the development and prevalence of AF in hypertensive patients have traditionally been taken from epidemiological data of patients with other comorbidities such as cardiac failure, valvular or coronary heart disease, and not uncomplicated hypertensive patients. Therefore historically this led to difficulties in risk stratifying hypertension as a

Box 10.1 Risk factors for atrial fibrillation
Hypertension
Age
Male gender
Coronary artery disease
Left atrial enlargement
Congestive cardiac disease
Left ventricular enlargement
Thyrotoxicosis
Valvular heart disease
Diabetes
Stroke
Smoking

potential protagonist of AF. Ciaroni and colleagues studied 97 initially untreated hypertensive patients, with an average age of 65 years, and found 19 developed AF during a 25-month follow-up period. The independent predictors were daytime and night-time ambulatory blood pressure, age, LV mass, LA dimensions, and peak velocity of A-wave on echocardiography. A similar study by Verdecchia and colleagues studied incidence, determinants, and outcomes of AF in a cohort of initially untreated hypertensive patients in sinus rhythm and the absence of valvular or coronary heart disease, thyroid, or lung disease. They noted that age and LV mass were the sole independent predictors of AF. Left atrial diameter was found to be an independent factor for AF after age and LV mass adjustments. Interestingly, LV mass and LA size were noted to be independent predictor of AF in apparently uncomplicated subjects with essential hypertension in both studies.

Left atrial dilation was noted to be a precursor of AF in the Framingham Heart Study and the Cardiovascular Health Study. Left atrial dilatation was shown to shorten refractory period and prolong conduction time, both factors that may contribute to formation of multiple re-entrant electrical circuits and therefore may propagate AF. Mattioli and colleagues found that patients with recurrence of AF after electrical cardioversion were more likely to have a larger left atrium and a smaller A-wave on echocardiography post cardioversion. LA size has been linked to systolic blood pressure and LVH in older patients with isolated hypertension. LV mass has been thought to reflect the cumulative long-term effects of haemodynamic factors that may exert detrimental effects on cardiovascular system. Therefore it is perhaps not surprising that LV mass has become recognized as a strong predictive factor of cardiovascular complications in the general population but especially in hypertensive patients.

10.2 **Pathophysiology**

There have been several different pathophysiological mechanisms that have been postulated to the development of AF in hypertensive patients. These include structural changes, neuro-endocrine activation and myocardial fibrosis. Suboptimally treated long-standing hypertension may lead to LVH with subsequent structural changes; for example, LA enlargement, changes in atrial conduction pathways, and fibrosis. These may contribute to the development of atrial fibrillation.

LVH can be interpreted as a manifestation of subclinical organ damage as a consequence of untreated or suboptimally treated HTN and is considered to be one of the most significant independent risk factor for AF. LVH reduces LV compliance and therefore increasing LV stiffness

Table 10.1 Myocardial remodelling attributed to predispose to the development of AF

Remodelling feature	Mechanism
Electrical	Reduction in action potential due to changes in intracellular calcium handling in both AF and PAF. This is potentially a reversible phenomenon on restoration of sinus rhythm.
Contractile	Changes in calcium handling due to micro re-entrant circuits result in reduction of effective atria contraction leading to stasis of blood within atria and therefore promoting haemostasis with subsequent increased risk of thrombo-embolic stroke.
Structural	Decrease in LV systolic function due to micro and macroscopic changes within the myocardium

which in turn leads to increased LV filling pressure and wall stress. Subsequently this results in activation of the sympathetic and renin–angiotensin–aldosterone system. The increased LV filling pressures result in increased atrial pressures resulting in dilated atria. The fibroblasts of the enlarged atria subsequently differentiate into myofibroblasts that enhance connective tissue deposition and fibrosis. The structural remodelling that results from deposition of fibrous tissue causes disruption between the myocytes, and electrical bundles potentiates the formation of multiple micro re-entrant circuits that are the pathognomonic of AF. AF may alter intracellular calcium handling (Table 10.1). This remodelling not only further perpetuates but also stabilizes AF micro re-entrant electrical currents, therefore giving rise to the phrase 'AF begets AF'.

10.3 **Treatment strategies**

There are a number of drugs that have been used to treat patients with hypertension and AF. These include angiotensin-converting enzyme inhibitors and angiotensin receptor blockers, beta blockers, and calcium channel blockers. Certain antihypertensive medications may reduce the risk of AF by lowering blood pressure but also by mechanisms described below.

10.3.1 **Angiotensin-converting enzyme inhibitors and angiotensin receptor blockers**

Angiotensin-converting enzyme inhibitors (ACE-I) and angiotensin receptor blockers (ARB) are commonly used in the treatment of hypertension. Some studies, however, have suggested a beneficial role in both prevention and management of AF in certain subgroups of patients. The beneficial effects of ACE-I and ARBs in reducing the incidence of AF in hypertensive patients are thought to be mediated by the prevention of left atrial enlargement, development of myocardial fibrosis, and LV dysfunction.

A meta-analysis of 11 studies by Healy and colleagues noted a 28% (range of 15–40%), relative risk reduction in the onset of new AF with the use of ACE-I. However, this effect was limited to patients with LVH or systolic dysfunction. Similarly, a meta-analysis by Schneider and colleagues found a 32% reduction in the incidence of AF for both ACE-I- and ARB-treated patients. The ONTARGET study also noted no difference in the incidence of new-onset AF between an ARB (telmisartan) or ACE-I (ramipril) treated patients. Primary prevention of AF was seen in patients with LVH or cardiac failure. The meta-analysis also noted a reduced odds for recurrence of AF after electrical cardioversion by 45%. The trials mentioned in the meta-analysis where not primary AF trials. Kalus and colleagues found ACE-I and ARBs were associated with a relative risk reduction of new-onset AF by 49%, a 53% reduction in failure rate of electrical cardioversion, and a 61% reduction in recurrence of AF after electrical cardioversion in patients with recent congestive cardiac failure. The VALUE trial showed valsartan associated with a 16% reduction in the incidence of at least one documented occurrence of new-onset AF but also a reduction in the incidence of persistent atrial fibrillation by 32% when compared to amlodipine. The study also found losartan was superior to atenolol in reducing the incidence of new-onset AF.

The TRANSCEND and the PROFESS trials found no protective effect of ARB against AF. The Heart Outcomes Prevention Evaluation study looked at patients known to have a number of cardiovascular risk factors, importantly with no LVH, impaired systolic function, or cardiac failure. The patients were then randomized into two treatment groups, ACE-I (ramipril), or a placebo. The study noted no significant difference in the development of AF. The CAPRAF study failed to demonstrate any benefit of the use of ARB (candesartan) for the preservation of sinus rhythm after electrical cardioversion in patients who did not receive antiarrhythmic drug therapy. Moreover the GISSI-AF study with 1442 patients, including 85% of patients with hypertension, who had either PAF or recently electrically cardioverted AF showed that ARB (valsartan) conferred no benefit on maintenance of sinus rhythm even in patients on optimal medical therapy, including antiarrhythmic drugs and ACE-I on the time to first AF recurrence.

In patients with cardiac failure, ARBs such as losartan and valsartan appear to confer greater prevention of first occurrence of AF than either beta blockers or calcium-channel blockers in hypertensive patients with LVH. However ARBs have not been shown to prevent recurrence of paroxysmal atrial fibrillation (PAF) or persistent AF. Therefore, the use of ARBs in preventing AF is limited to those hypertensive patients with LVH or impaired systolic function. The ACTIVE I trial found that irbesartan (an ARB) had no beneficial effect in high-risk patients with ischaemic heart disease or in patients with persistent AF.

10.3.2 Beta blockers

Beta blockers are not routinely recommended as first-line treatment in uncomplicated hypertension. However, they still have a valuable role in treatment of patients with AF in terms of ventricular rate control but also maintenance of sinus rhythm, the latter perhaps by virtue of preventing reverse remodelling, decreasing sympathetic drive thereby decreasing ischaemic drive and shortening of the action potential, factors that may otherwise give rise to formation of micro re-entrant electrical circuits and therefore AF. Of special mention, sotalol, a non-selective beta blocker Class III anti-arrhythmic, has been noted to be particularly effective in maintaining sinus rhythm after electrical cardioversion. However, sotalol has recognized pro-arrhythmic effects such as that of prolongation of QTc interval and the consequent predisposition of ventricular arrhythmias. There is at present a lack of data suggesting the prevention of new-onset atrial fibrillation.

10.3.3 Calcium-channel blockers

This group of drugs includes agents with both antihypertensive properties—for example, amlodipine and felodipine—and it also includes non-dihydropyridines such as diltiazem and verapamil that are commonly used to control ventricular rate control in patients with AF. De Simone and colleagues noted that the addition of verapamil significantly reduced recurrence of AF within three months after electrical cardioversion when compared to patients being treated with propafenone alone. However, this was not reproduced in other studies. Amlodipine was inferior to valsartan in preventing new-onset AF in the VALUE trial. Furthermore, in a four-year American, follow-up retrospective study of almost 5500 patients from the National Integrated Medical and Pharmacy claims database that were treated for hypertension with either an ACE-I or calcium-channel blocker, noted that new-onset AF was significantly lower in the ACE-I group.

The UK GP research database consisting of 4661 patients with AF and 18 641 matched controlled hypertensive patients were compared. The study noted patients treated with ACE-I, ARBs, or beta bockers were associated with lower risk of AF than those patients treated with CCB. However, treatment bias could not be excluded.

Although therefore CCBs do not have a role in the prevention of AF in hypertensive patients, non-dihydropyridine calcium antagonists are recommended to control ventricular rate in AF patients, especially where beta blockers cannot be used.

10.3.4 **Thromboprophylaxis**

Finally, all patients with AF must have their risk of thrombo-embolic stroke assessed for treatment with formal anticoagulation. This is especially true of patients with concomitant hypertension. Hypertension is given a score of 1 in the CHADS$_2$VASC scoring system.

10.4 **Conclusion**

Hypertension is a common cardiovascular disorder. Hypertensive patients have also been noted to be at increased risk of the development of AF. In fact, hypertension is the most common disorder in atrial fibrillation trials. It is therefore not surprising that both hypertension and AF are thought to be inextricably linked. AF increases the overall mortality, stroke, heart failure, and hospitalization, and it affects quality of life. The co-existence of hypertension and atrial fibrillation has been reported to double the risk for all of the forementioned. The development of AF in hypertensive patients has been postulated to be secondary to atrial remodelling via electrical, contractile and structural changes within the atria. This emphasizes the importance of optimizing medical treatment strategies of hypertensive patients, thereby minimizing potential complications. Mainstay medical therapy consists of the use of beta blockers, drugs blocking renin–angiotensin–aldosterone system, and calcium-channel blockers. Drugs blocking the renin–angiotensin–aldosterone system reduces the risk of new-onset AF in patients with LVH, LV systolic dysfunction, and cardiac failure. Beta blockers are effective for rate control with certain beta blockers maintaining sinus rhythm. There is at present a lack of data suggesting the prevention of new-onset atrial fibrillation.

Key references

Benjamin EJ, Wolf PA, D'Agostino RB, *et al.* (1998). Impact of atrial fibrillation on the risk of death: the Framingham Heart Study. *Circulation*; 98:946–52.

Camm AJ, Lip GY, De Caterina R, *et al.* (2012). 2012 focused update of theESC Guidelines for the management of atrial fibrillation: An update of the 2010 ESC Guidelines for the management of atrial fibrillation. *European Heart Journal*; 33:2719–274.

Ciaroni S, Cuenoud L, Bloch A (2000). Clinical study to investigate the predictive parameters for the onset of atrial fibrillation in patients with essential hypertension. American *Heart Journal*; 139:814–19.

The Working Group on Hypertension, Arrhythmias and Thrombosis of the European Society of Hypertension (2012). Hypertension and atrial fibrillation: diagnostic approach, prevention and treatment. *Journal of Hypertension*; 2012, 30:239–52.

Kalus JS, Coleman CI, White CM (2006). The impact of suppressing the reninangiotensin system on atrial fibrillation. *Journal of Clinical Pharmacology*; 46:21–8.

Kirchhof P, Lip GY, Van Gelder IC, *et al.* (2011). Comprehensive risk reduction in patients with atrial fibrillation: Emerging diagnostic and therapeutic options. Executive summary of the report from the 3rd AFNET/EHRA consensus conference. *Thrombosis Haemostasis*; 106:1012–19.

Manolis AJ, Rosei EA, Coca A, Cifkova R, et al. (2012). Hypertension and atrial fibrillation: diagnostic approach, prevention and treatment. Position paper of the Working Group 'Hypertension Arrhythmias and Thrombosis' of the European Society of Hypertension. *Journal of Hypertension*; 30:239–52.

Schaer BA, Schneider C, Jick SS (2010). Risk for incident atrial fibrillation in patients who receive antihypertensive drugs: a nested case-control study. *Annals of Internal Medicine*; 152:78–84.

Schneider MP, Hua TA, Bohm M, et al. (2010). Prevention of atrial fibrillation by renin-angiotensin system-inhibition a meta-analysis. *Journal of the American College of Cardiology*; 55:2299–307.

Verdecchia P, Reboldi G, Gattobigio R, et al. (2003). Atrial Fibrillation in Hypertension: Predictors and Outcome. *Hypertension*; 41:218–23.

Part 3

Management and treatment of hypertension

Chapter 11

Non-pharmacological management of hypertension

Kully Sandhu and Sunil Nadar

> ## Key points
>
> - Lifestyle modifications are an important part of hypertension management.
> - These changes help in lowering the overall cardiovascular risk along with blood pressure control.
> - Regular exercise with the maintenance of optimal body weight and a healthy diet complement pharmacologic treatment.
> - In most cases lifestyle modification on its own is not sufficient to control hypertension and requires pharmacologic intervention as well.

11.1 Introduction

The exact pathogenesis of primary hypertension is not fully understood. There is, however, growing evidence that lifestyle modification can significant reduce blood pressure not only in patients with established hypertension but also in those with prehypertension. Prospective meta-analysis of over a million adults aged 40–69 years had double the risk of death from coronary heart disease with each 20 mmHg and 10 mmHg increase in baseline systolic and diastolic blood pressures respectively.

Many controlled trials and population-based studies have underpinned the importance of lifestyle changes as an integral part of lowering blood pressure in both hypertensive and prehypertensive patients. Indeed, some studies have seen lifestyle changes to be as effective as a single antihypertensive agent in lowering blood pressure. Despite lifestyle modifications appearing to offer only incremental reduction in blood pressure—by 5 mmHg in observational studies—these have been associated with reductions in mortality by stroke, heart disease, and all-cause mortality by 14%, 9%, and 7% respectively. This had led to the Seventh Report of the Joint National Committee on Prevention, Detection, Evaluation and Treatment of High Blood Pressure recommendations not to discontinue recommending lifestyle modifications (Table 11.1). In some patients, stringent non-pharmacological measures may occasionally allow reduction in or cessation of drug therapy. The 2011 guidelines of the British Hypertension Society (BHS) urge that non-pharmacological measures be used in all hypertensive patients.

11.2 Primary prevention

Although it is not clear to what extent lifestyle modifications help in the primary prevention of hypertension, population studies suggest that many lifestyle changes help prevent the rise of

Table 11.1 Effect of non pharmacological and lifestyle modifications on blood pressure

Modification	Comment
Maintain ideal body weight/weight reduction	Blood pressure reduced by 5–10 mmHg for each 10 kg weight loss
Aerobic physical exercise	May reduce blood pressure by as much as 13/8 mmHg
Diet rich in fruits and vegetables, low-fat dairy products, reduced intake of saturated fats	Up to 11/5 mmHg reduction in eight weeks
Sodium intake limited to 100 mmol per day (6 g of sodium chloride)	Lowers blood pressure by 4/2 mmHg
At least 90 mmol of dietary potassium a day	
Adequate dietary calcium and magnesium	
Limit alcohol to 23 units per week (19 units for women)	Lowers blood pressure by up to 4/2 mmHg
Smoking cessation	

blood pressure with age and therefore reduce the prevalence of hypertension in the overall population. The recommendations as outlined by the British Hypertension Society include the following:

• Maintenance of normal body weight

• Decrease in dietary sodium intake to < 6 g of salt a day

• Regular aerobic physical activity

• Limit alcohol consumption to no more than three units/day in men and two units/day in women

• Diet rich in fruit and vegetables

• Diet with reduced content of saturated and total fat

11.3 **Dietary changes**

Diet is one of the main distinguishing factors of a particular community and therefore could have a bearing on the different blood pressure profiles. For example, studies have shown lower blood pressure in countries where there are large populations which adhere to either vegetarian or vegan diets. This phenomenon can also be seen in communities that have a predominantly vegetarian or vegan diet in industrialized.

There are epidemiological studies suggesting the Mediterranean diet, rich in olive oil, is associated with lower blood pressure. In cross-over trials, olive oil has been associated with lower blood pressure when compared with sunflower oil supplements. Olive oil is rich in monounsaturated fatty acids and oleic acid whereas sunflower and other vegetable oils are rich in polyunsaturated fatty acids and linoleic acids. Therefore it has been proposed that diets rich in monounsaturated fatty acids may be effective in lowering blood pressure. Other possible mechanisms involved could include the fact that extra-virgin olive oil is rich in antioxidant polyphenols, which are totally absent in vegetable oils.

More recently the INTERMAP study (International Study of Macro- and Micro-nutrients and Blood Pressure), an international epidemiologic study of 4680 men and women aged 40–59 from China, Japan, the United Kingdom, and United States, found that diets rich in vegetable

Table 11.2 Dietary advice	
High	Low
Fruit and vegetables (four or five portions /day)	Saturated fat
Fiber	Cholesterol
Low fat dairy products (two to three servings a day)	Low-sodium salt
Lean meat (two or three portions a day)	
Calcium	
Magnesium	
Potassiun	

proteins and omega-3 polyunsaturated fats could help not only prevent but may also control high blood pressure (see Table 11.2).

Currently the use of vitamin C, coenzyme Q10, and magnesium in management of hypertension is not recommended due of the lack of data from well-designed randomized controlled trials.

11.4 **Dietary salt**

Over the last thousand years the human diet has changed as a consequence of salt used in food preservation and preparation. The resultant dietary potassium-to-sodium ratio has consequently reduced by a factor of 100–200. This is based on the comparison of the modern diet with that of the Yanomamos, tribe of Amazonian rainforest Indians. The Yanomamos have been labelled as the 'no-salt culture' by virtue of the fact they consume very little sodium salt and consume a largely vegetarian potassium diet. There was no increase in blood pressure (BP) with age and hypertension was virtually absent.

There are a number of clinical trials and epidemiologic studies that implicate increased sodium intake with increase not only in blood pressure but also reduced incidence of cardiovascular events (Trials of Hypertension Prevention, TOHP). One of the largest epidemiological study was the International Cooperative Study on the Relation of Sodium and Potassium to Blood Pressure (INTERSALT). INTERSALT investigated the relation of urine sodium excretion to blood pressure and included over 10 000 men and women from over 32 countries. The study found a highly significant relationship between sodium intake and blood pressure. They noted a systolic and diastolic decrease in blood pressure of 10–12 mmHg and 6–7 mmHg respectively with a population median sodium decreased by 100 mmol per day. The study also concluded that habitual high sodium intake together with low potassium intake, reduced physical activity, high BMI, and excess alcohol intake are important environmental factors in the prevalence of hypertension.

Several randomized placebo controlled studies have also recommended an upper limit for sodium intake of 2300 mg per day, corresponding to approximately 6 grams of salt per day. The exact pathophysiological mechanism that increased sodium intake increases blood pressure still remains unclear, however it is postulated that increased sodium causes fluid retention which causes fluid overload, thereby increasing blood pressure. The main problem with low-salt diets is strict compliance by patients. Interestingly, only 20% of hypertensive patients were compliant with low-sodium diets, as measured by urinary sodium excretion < 75 mmol/day. Low-sodium salt substitutes may be used, but these are potassium based and thus can be associated with a higher incidence of hyperkalaemia, and therefore should be avoided in patients on potassium-sparing diuretics. Salt intake is a public health priority both at an individual and population level. At the individual level, effective salt reduction is by no means easy to achieve. Advice should be given to avoid added salt and high-salt food. However, sodium reduction at population level may be even more difficult to achieve because as much as 80% of salt consumption may be consumed as hidden salt within processed bread, meat, cheese, margarine, and cereals.

11.5 **Weight reduction**

There is a strong association between obesity and hypertension. Several studies have shown that a reduction in systolic and diastolic pressures occurs with weight loss. A meta-analysis of 11 studies showed that a 1 kg reduction in body weight causes a reduction of blood pressure. A Cochrane review of six randomized trials showed that a weight loss in the range of 4–8% was associated with a decrease in blood pressure in the range of 3 mmHg for both systolic and diastolic blood pressure.

11.6 **Potassium**

The INTERSALT trial demonstrated an association of higher levels of urinary potassium excretion with lower blood pressures. Diets rich in fruits and vegetables have a high potassium content, which could explain their benefit. The exact mechanism behind this is not clear, however we know that sodium and potassium act antagonistically such that a decrease in potassium results in sodium retention and this leads to increased intravascular volume and therefore higher blood pressure. An increased intake of potassium tends to promote sodium excretion and therefore diuresis with subsequent decrease in blood pressure. It has been suggested that in patients with essential hypertension, a diet low in potassium resulted in a systolic blood pressure increase of 7 mmHg was due to sodium retention. There is good evidence to suggest that increasing potassium intake with a diet rich in fruits and vegetables does lower blood pressure and therefore helps to prevent strokes. The high potassium content of fruits and vegetables could play a role in reducing blood pressure, possibly by the natriuretic effect that potassium is thought to have. Increasing the potassium content in the diet may also have the added benefits of anti-oxidants and vitamins that fruits and vegetables have. However, the role of potassium supplementation in hypertension is uncertain, with different trials showing conflicting results. Cappuccio and colleagues conducted meta-analyses on 19 trials involving 586 patients of whom 412 had essential hypertension. The meta-analysis suggested that oral potassium supplements significantly lowered mean systolic and diastolic blood pressure by 5.9 mmHg and 3.4 mmHg respectively. Interestingly, the greatest reduction in blood pressure appeared to be in patients with hypertension, and this seemed to be more pronounced the longer the potassium supplementation was given. The group thus recommended that potassium should be included in the strategy for non-pharmacological management for hypertension. Great caution in potassium supplementation is required in many patients who have renal impairment or patients on potassium-sparing diuretics. Current recommendations are to obtain adequate potassium intake through a healthy diet.

11.7 **Coffee drinking**

There currently is no general consensus of the effect of caffeine, with conflicting evidence in the literature and with the effects of caffeine depending on several variables such as the daily dose, coffee-drinking habits, and patients' pre-existing blood pressure. However ingestion of 250 mg of caffeine appears to be associated with an increase of 6 mmHg and 10 mmHg increase in systolic blood pressure in normotensive and hypertensive patients respectively. Similarly, a 5 mmHg and 8.5 mmHg increase in diastolic blood pressure in controls and hypertensive patients respectively. A meta-analysis of 11 trials showed that chronic coffee drinkers (average of five cups/day) have blood pressure values slightly higher than non-drinkers. However, there are currently no trials that have assessed the effect of the cessation of drinking coffee on blood pressure in hypertensive patients.

11.8 **Alcohol**

The association between alcohol and high blood pressure is well documented both in population and clinical studies. However, studies involving alcohol must be viewed with caution, as it is likely that patients consuming large quantities of alcohol are very unlikely to be involved in clinical trials. Individuals tend to under-report alcohol consumption. Finally, patterns of alcohol consumption, type of alcohol consumed, etc., depends to a large extent on socio-economic factors, many of which may not be corrected for in the analysis.

An alcohol intake of around 80 g per day (equivalent to four pints of beer) has been shown to raise blood pressure, particularly in hypertensive patients. Alcohol also increases the risk of cardiomyopathy and atrial fibrillation. Blood pressure tends to fall when alcohol is stopped or reduced, and remains low in those patients who continue to abstain. A systematic review and a meta-analysis of alcohol intervention studies have shown that alcohol restriction reduces systolic and diastolic blood pressure by 2.7 mmHg and 1.4 mmHg, respectively.

There are conflicting data on what constitutes 'safe' alcohol consumption levels in hypertension. In the Physicians Health Study cohort, it was found that compared with individuals who reported that they rarely or never drank alcohol, those who reported monthly, weekly, or daily consumption had increasingly significant trends for reduced total and cardiovascular mortality. The beneficial effects of light to moderate drinking were seen regardless of whether blood pressure levels were above or below 140/90 mmHg. It was also shown that consumption of as little as a single alcoholic drink monthly could reduce overall cardiovascular risk by 18%. This strongly suggests the results being confounded by an unmeasured factor. A similar study from France that involved a 13- to 21-year follow-up of 36 583 initially healthy middle-aged men showed that moderate wine drinkers (< 60 g alcohol/day) had lower risks of deaths from all causes at all levels of systolic blood pressure. No significant reduction in all-cause mortality was seen in heavier drinkers or in those who consumed beer or spirits predominantly. Again, the presence of a significant confounder appears very likely. A substudy of the Losartan Intervention For Endpoint reduction in hypertension (LIFE) study found that in drinkers there was no decrease in composite cardiovascular risk when being treated with losartan compared with atenolol because a decrease in the incidence of myocardial infarction in the drinkers was offset by an increase in the risk of stroke.

The Prevention and Treatment of Hypertension Study (PATHS) found that alcohol cessation in hypertensive patients had a 1.2/0.7 mmHg greater reduction in BP than the control group at the end of a six-month period. This was, however, non-significant. Hypertensive men who drink alcohol should be advised to limit their consumption to no more than 20–30 g, and hypertensive women to no more than 10–20 g, of alcohol per day. Total alcohol consumption should not exceed 140 g per week for men and 80 g per week for women. A meta-analysis of studies looking at the effect of alcohol on blood pressure showed an overall statistically significant reduction in blood pressure with a three-drinks/day reduction in alcohol consumption leading to reductions in blood pressure. There were reductions of 3 mmHg in systolic blood pressure and 2 mmHg in diastolic blood pressure for patients in the alcohol reduction groups (average reduction of 67% from an average intake of three to six drinks per day at baseline).

A reduction by one drink/day in moderate-to-heavy drinkers led to an approximately 1 mmHg reduction in blood pressure. Although this may seem modest it does represent a substantial improvement in blood pressure profile overall.

The Seventh Report of the Joint National Committee on the prevention, detection, evaluation, and treatment of high blood pressure (JNC-7) recommends no more than two drinks of alcohol a day for men and one drink a day for women or men of lighter build. The Fourth British Hypertension Society (BHS-IV) recommends not more than three units a day for men and two units a day for women as primary prevention of hypertension, and in patients with established hypertension, they recommend not more than 21 units a week for men and 14 units a week for women. They suggest that limiting to this level of alcohol consumption could reduce blood pressures by 2–4 mmHg.

11.9 **Conclusion**

Epidemiological data support contribution of several dietary and other lifestyle-related factors to the development of high blood pressure. The PREMIER trial studied 810 patients with established hypertension and then randomized to one of three groups. The first group underwent strict lifestyle modifications (limiting salt and alcohol intake, increasing physical activity, and weight reduction); the second group underwent the same but also adhered to the 'Dietary Approach to Stop Hypertension' DASH diet. The DASH diet was rich in potassium, magnesium, and calcium. It was also rich in whole grains, poultry, fish, and nuts whilst being low in red meat, sweets, and sugar-containing beverages. The third group were only given advice about lifestyle modifications and they were not strictly monitored. There was a significant decrease in blood pressure in the groups with strict lifestyle modifications, the maximum reduction being in the group who modified their lifestyle and followed the DASH diet. This trial was one of the first studies to look at all the lifestyle factors together, not simply individual factors in isolation, and it underlined the importance of ensuring that patients follow lifestyle modifications.

Non-pharmacological based advice is an essential and integral part of managing not only hypertension but also in reducing overall cardiovascular mortality and morbidity. The importance of physical activity, reduction of body weight, sodium salt intake, alcohol, and perhaps coffee consumption should be emphasized. However, the main obstacle remains patient compliance. Therefore, all treating physicians must spend time with patients to explain the importance of non-pharmacological modifications.

Key references

Appel LJ, Champagne CM, Harsha DW, et al. (2003). Effects of comprehensive lifestyle modification on blood pressure control: main results of the PREMIER clinical trial. Journal of American Medical Association; 289(16): 2083–93.

Beasley JM, Ange B, Anderson CAM, et al. (2009). Associations Between Macronutrient Intake and Self-reported Appetite and Fasting Levels of Appetite Hormones: Results From the Optimal Macronutrient Intake Trial to Prevent Heart Disease. American Journal of Epidemiology; 169 (7): 893-900. doi: 10.1093/aje/kwn415.

Cappuccio FP, MacGregor GA (1991). Does potassium supplementation reduce blood pressure: A meta-analysis of randomised trials. Journal of Hypertension; 9(5): 465–73.

Cook NR, Cutler JA, Obarzanek E, et al. (2007). Long term effects of dietary sodium reduction on cardiovascular disease outcomes: observational follow-up of the trials of hypertension prevention (TOHP). BMJ; 334: 885–88.

Geleijnse JM, Kok FJ, Grobbee DE (2003). Blood pressure response to changes in sodium and potassium intake: a metaregression analysis of randomized trials. Journal of Human Hypertension; 17: 471-80.

Gallen IW, Rosa RM, Esparaz DY, *et al.* (1998). On the mechanism of the effects of potassium restriction on blood pressure and renal sodium retention. *American Journal of Kidney Disease*; 31: 19-27.

NICE Hypertension Guidelines. <http://guidance.nice.org.uk/CG127>

Sachs FM, Svetkey LP, Vollmer WM, *et al.* (2001). Effects on blood pressure of reduced dietary sodium and the Dietary Approaches to Stop Hypertension (DASH) diet. DASH- sodium collaborative Research Group. *New England Journal of Medicine*; 344(1):3–10.

Stamler J, Rose G, Stamler R, *et al.* (1989). INTERSALT study findings. Public health and medical care implications. *Hypertension*; 14(5): 570–77.

Chobanian AV, Bakris GL, Black HR, *et al.* (2003). Seventh report of the Joint National Committee on Prevention, Detection, Evaluation, and Treatment of High Blood Pressure. *Hypertension*; 42: 1206–52.

Chapter 12

Diuretics in hypertension

Mehmood Sadiq Butt

Key points

- Diuretics are effective both as sole agents and as combination agents with other antihypertensive drugs. The choice of agent will depend on various factors including age, ethnicity, and presence of comorbidities.
- Loop diuretics are more effective than thiazide diuretics in advanced renal failure.
- Rigorous monitoring of electrolyte balance and renal function is essential during treatment.
- Combination of thiazide or loop diuretics with a potassium-sparing agent may further improve blood pressure control and aid maintenance of normokalaemia.

12.1 Introduction

Diuretics continue to play an important role in the treatment of hypertension. In addition, they remain the cornerstone of treatment of congestive cardiac failure, liver failure (ascities), and renal failure. Cost-effectiveness, high compliance, and evidence from early studies have meant that diuretics have had a consistent track record in the treatment of both newly diagnosed and refractory hypertension.

12.2 Classification of diuretics

On the basis of their mechanism and site of action in the nephron (Figure 12.1), diuretics can be broadly classified into three major sub-classes:

- Thiazide diuretics
- Loop-acting diuretics
- Potassium-sparing diuretics

12.3 Thiazide diuretics

Thiazides are used to treat hypertension and congestive cardiac failure. The 2011 UK National institute of Health and Care Excellence (NICE) recommends adding thiazide diuretics to angiotensin-converting enzyme inhibitors or calcium-channel blockers (NICE guidelines, GC 127). They control hypertension by blocking the thiazide-sensitive Na^+/Cl^- pump in the distal convoluted tubule of the nephrons and hence prevent re-absorption of sodium and chloride ions (Figure 12.1). Thiazides have favourable pharmacokinetic profile and reach peak levels within 2–6 hours of ingestion (Table 12.1).

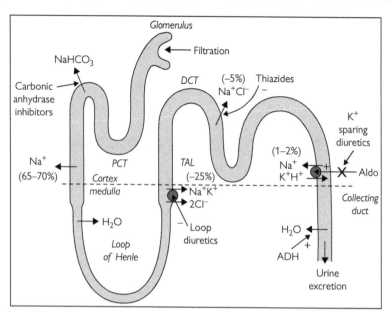

Figure 12.1 Diaphragmatic representation of the nephron depicting sites of action of the three major classes of diuretics

PCT, proximal convoluted tubule; TAL, thick ascending limb; DCT, distal convoluted tubule; Aldo, aldosterone; ADH, anti-diuretic hormone.

Table 12.1 Pharmacokinetics of thiazide diuretics		
Diuretic	% Oral bioavailability	Elimination half-life (hours)
Bendroflumethiazide (2.5–5 mg/day; mane)	ND	2–5
Chlortalidone (25–50 mg/day; mane)	64	24–55
Hydrochlorthiazide (12.5–25 mg/day; mane)	65–75	2.5
Indapamide (2.5 mg/day; mane)	92	15–25
ND: Not determined		

12.3.1 Contraindications

• Hypersensitivity to thiazides or sulfonamides
• Lithium therapy (bipolar disorder)
• Pregnancy and breastfeeding
• Severe renal impairment

12.3.2 **Adverse effects**

- Metabolic disturbances
  - Hypokalemia (concurrent ACE inhibitor may balance this)
  - Hyponatremia (can cause confusion in extreme cases)
  - Hypercalcemia (little clinical significance)
  - Hyperuricemia (can cause gout)
  - Hypovolemia
  - Metabolic alkalosis
- Gastrointestinal
  - Anorexia, jaundice, pancreatitis, and hepatic coma (should be stopped)
- Blood discrasias
  - Leukopaenia, agranulocytosis, thrombocytopaenia, aplastic anaemia, and hamemolytic anemia
- Other
  - Orthostatic hypotension (common, in particular amongst the elderly. If there is a significant drop in systolic blood pressure upon standing, the dose should be reduced or the agent stopped until asymptomatic).
  - Acute interstitial pneumonitis (rare, but can be life-threatening).
  - Hyperglycemia, in particular when used with beta-adrenergic receptor blockers.

12.3.3 **Interactions**

A detailed treatise of drug interactions is outside the scope of this text, but care is advisable when prescribing thiazide diuretics with oral anticoagulants, steroids, and lithium (lithium toxicity may rapidly develop).

12.3.4 **Indications**

NICE recommends addition of thiazide-like diuretic in step 3 or 4 (when a combination of ACE inhibitor and calcium-channel blocker is already in use) in the four-step cascade for the management of hypertension in patients of any age or ethnicity (NICE 2011 guidelines, GC 127).

Metolazone (2.5–5 mg/day) is a particularly potent thiazide-like diuretic that acts both on the early part of the distal and proximal convoluted tubules. Literature review suggests that combination with loop diuretics in patients with congestive cardiac failure increases urine output and improves clinical profile (Rosenberg et al.).

Indapamide (2.5 mg/day; mane) is another well-studied diuretic that is used for the treatment of hypertension. In the recent Action in Diabetes and Vascular disease: Preterax and Diamicron MR controlled Evaluation (ADVANCE) study, a combination of indapamide and perindopril, when given to diabetic subjects, was shown to reduce the risk of a micro- or macrovascular event by 9%.

12.4 **Loop diuretics**

These rapidly acting agents are available in both oral and intravenous preparations. They are mostly used in the treatment of heart failure and are more efficacious in subjects with impaired renal profile compared with thiazides (which are more effective in patients with normal renal functions).

12.4.1 **Mechanism of action**

Loop diuretics exert their action by blocking the $Na^+/K^+/Cl^-$ transport system in the thick part of the ascending loop of Henle (Figure 12.1). This results in increased luminal concentration of Na^+, K^+, Mg^{2+}, and Ca^{2+} and consequently fluid diuresis. In addition to this, they also enhance prostaglandin-mediated venodilatation thereby resulting in fluid redistribution and reducing cardiac preload, thus improving the symptoms of cardiac failure.

12.4.2 **Contraindications, adverse effects and drug interactions**

- As with thiazide diuretics, the most common side effects relate to excessive diuresis and metabolic disturbance. Hypokalaemia, hypocalcaemia, hypomagnesaemia, and hypochloraemic can all occur.
- Use of loop diuretics should be avoided in pregnancy (teratogenicity), hepatic failure, hypokalaemia, hypotension, and drug hypersensitivity.
- Hyperosmolar non-ketotic coma can be precipitated in diabetics, and agranulocytosis may rarely occur.
- Furosemide reduces the threshold for nephrotoxicity caused by aminoglycosides and cephalosporins when used concomitantly. It may also increase serum lithium levels and rapidly precipitate toxicity.

12.4.3 **Indications**

Furosemide (20–500 mg/day) is indicated in the treatment of heart failure. Intravenous preparations are generally used for decompensated cardiac failure, but can sometimes be considered for emergency treatment of blood pressure in hypertensive crises—although most authorities now recommend alternatives. In contrast to thiazide diuretics, loop diuretics retain their efficacy in renal failure and are used in such patients for controlling both hypertension and fluid balance, although substantially higher doses (up to 500 mg/day) may be required in the setting of renal failure and oliguria (e.g. max 2 g/day).

12.5 **Potassium-sparing diuretics and mineralocorticoid (aldosterone) antagonists**

Spironolactone, the aldosterone receptor antagonist; eplerenone, a selective mineralocorticoid receptor antagonist; and amiloride, an epithelial sodium-channel (ENaC) blocker are all very weak diuretics but are better known for their potassium-sparing effects. They have an important role to play in the treatment of heart failure, refractory hypertension, and also in portal hypertension secondary to liver cirrhosis.

12.5.1 **Mechanism of action**

In response to reduced renal perfusion ensuing from decreased cardiac output, hypotension, or ischaemia the juxtaglomerular cells increase secretion of renin (Figure 12.2). In addition, enhanced Na^+ diuresis and beta-adrenergic stimulation can both increase renin secretion. Renin converts angiotensiongen to angiotensin I. This in turn is converted to the potent vasoconstrictor, angiotensin II, by angiotensin-converting enzyme in the lungs. Angiotensin II stimulates aldosterone secretion by the adrenal glands. Aldosterone is a vasoconstrictor, enhances sodium resorption and promotes potassium excretion.

Spironolactone inhibits the aldosterone receptors located in the collecting tubule resulting in decreased reabsorption of Na^+ and reduced excretion of K^+ helping in diuresis while retaining K^+. The other potassium-sparing agents, amiloride and triamterene, interact with lumen

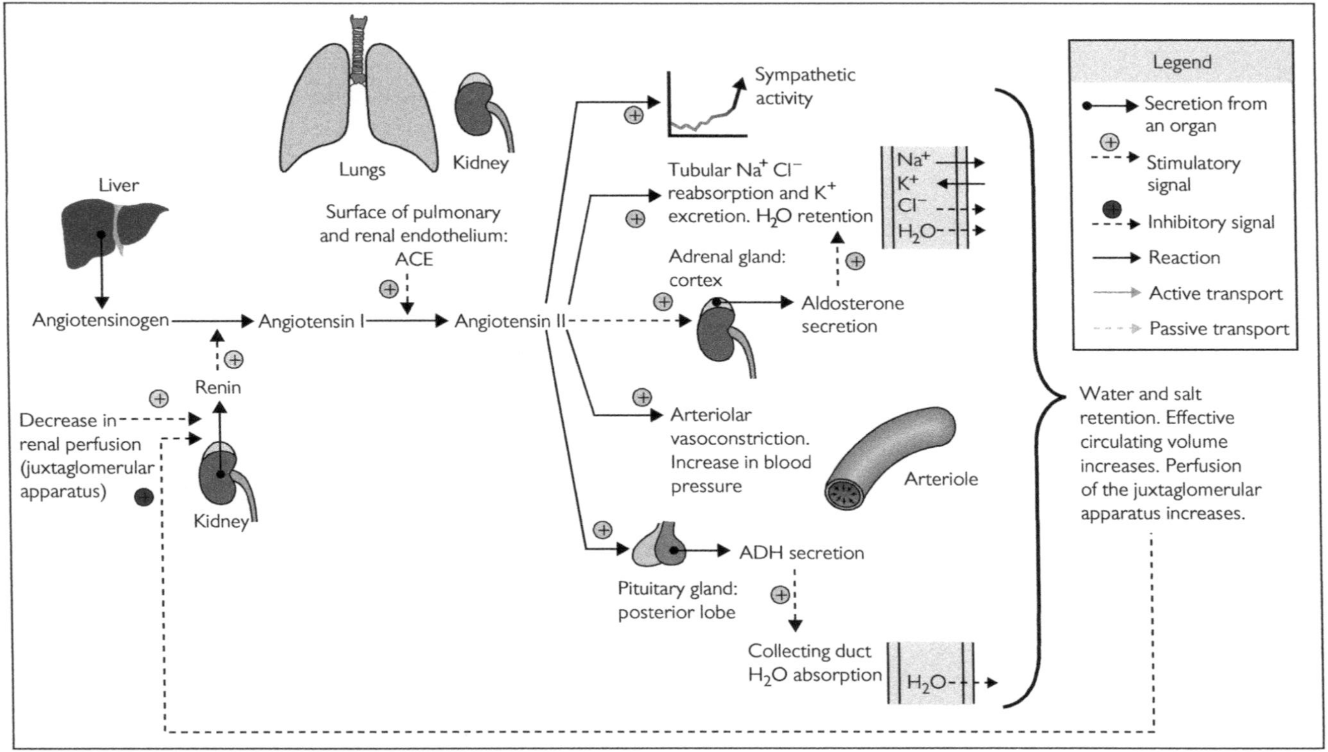

Figure 12.2 The renin–angiotensin–aldosterone cascade

ACE, angiotensin-converting enzyme; ADH, anti-diuretic hormone.

membrane transporters to prevent urinary Na^+ entry into the cytoplasm. They are both direct inhibitors of K^+ secretion.

12.5.2 Contraindications, adverse effects, and interactions

- Metabolic disturbances such as hyperkalemia and hyponatremia are not uncommon. Regular monitoring is advisable.
- Gynaecomastia in men (which may be painful) and menstrual irregularities in perimenopausal women are relatively common side effects with spironolactone.
- Triamterene is contraindicated in patients with a history of renal calculi as it precipitates calculus formation, although other potassium-sparing diuretics do not appear to cause this effect. In addition, concomitant use of NSAIDs and triamterene is best avoided as this precipitates renal failure.
- Best avoided if creatinine clearance is less than 20 ml/min.
- Aspirin may antagonize the effects of spironolactone.

12.5.3 Indications and uses

- NICE recommends addition of spironolactone in the fourth step of the management cascade (NICE guidelines, GC 127). RALES study demonstrated prognostic implications of spironolactone in advanced heart failure (Pitt et al.). Eplerenone, a more selective mineralocorticoid antagonist, has also shown beneficial effects on the long-term survival in patients with heart failure post myocardial infarction (EPHESUS study). It is recommended as a third- or fourth-line agent for use in resistant hypertension and in patients with significant side effects to spironolactone.
- By virtue of their mode of action, aldosterone antagonists used alone have very weak antihypertensive effects and therefore used as add-on with other antihypertension agent.
- Primary hyperaldosteronism is increasingly appreciated as an important cause of resistant hypertension. The addition of an aldosterone antagonist helps block the effects of excess aldosterone in these patients and frequently improves blood pressure. However, in such cases it remains important to assess for presence of an aldosterone-producing (Conn's) adenoma as this may require surgical intervention.
- Aldosterone antagonists are also valuable in treatment of metabolic disturbances (e.g. Liddle's and Bartter's syndromes), portal hypertension with ascites, and moderate-to-severe cardiac failure.

12.6 Summary

Diuretics continue to play an important and multifaceted role in the treatment of hypertension. Wide availability, cost-effectiveness, and a favourable safety profile ensure high compliance, whether used alone or as combination therapy. Importantly, the diuretics may have significant role in the management for other coexisting conditions such as congestive cardiac failure and some causes of secondary hypertension (e.g. hyperaldosteronism).

Key references

Brater DC (1998). Diuretic therapy. *New England Journal of Medicine*;339: 387.

Brown MJ, Palmer CR, Castaigne A, et al. (2000). Morbidity and mortality in patients randomised to double-blind treatment with a long-acting calcium-channel blocker or diuretic in the International Nifedipine GITS study: Intervention as a Goal in Hypertension Treatment (INSIGHT). *Lancet*; 356: 366–72.

Ettinger B, Oldroyd NO, Sorgel F (1980). Triamterene nephrolithiasis. *Journal of American Medical Association;* 244: 2443.

Favre L, Glasson P, Vallotton MB (1982). Reversible acute renal failure from combined triamterene and indomethacin: A study in healthy subjects. *Annals of Internal Medicines;* 96: 317.

Higgins B, Williams B, Guideline Development Group. (2007). Pharmacological management of hypertension. *Clinical Medicine;* 7: 612–6.

Juurlink DN, Mamdani MM, Kopp A, et al. (2004). Drug-induced lithium toxicity in the elderly: a population-based study. *Journal of American Geriatric Society;* 52: 794–8.

Kostis JB, Wilson AC, Freudenberger RS, et al. (2005). Long-term effect of diuretic-based therapy on fatal outcomes in subjects with isolated systolic hypertension with and without diabetes. *American Journal of Cardiology;* 95: 29–35.

Krakoff LR (2005). Diuretics for hypertension. *Circulation;* 112: e127–9.

NICE guidelines, GC 127. http://www.nice.org.uk/nicemedia/live/13561/56015/56015.pdf>

Pitt B, Zannad F, Remme WJ, et al. (1999). The effect of spironolactone on morbidity and mortality in patients with severe heart failure. Randomized Aldactone Evaluation Study Investigators. *New England Journal of Medicine.* 341:709–17

Rosenberg J, Gustafsson F, Galatius S, et al. (2005). Combination therapy with metolazone and loop diuretics in outpatients with refractory heart failure: an observational study and review of the literature. *Cardiovascular Drugs Therapy;*19: 301–6

Rossignol P, Ménard J, Fay R, et al. (2011). Eplerenone survival benefits in heart failure patients post-myocardial infarction are independent from its diuretic and potassium-sparing effects. Insights from an EPHESUS (Eplerenone Post-Acute Myocardial Infarction Heart Failure Efficacy and Survival Study) substudy. *Journal of the American College of Cardiology* 58: 1958–66.

Siscovick DS, Raghanathan TE, Psaty BM, et al. (1994). Diuretic therapy for hypertension and the risk of primary cardiac arrest. *New England Journal of Medicine;* 330: 1852.

Tamargo J, Sequra J, Ruilope LM (2014). Diuretics in the treatment of hypertension Part 2: loop diuretics and potassium sparring agents. *Expert Opinion in Pharmacotherapeutics;* 15:605–21.

Weinberger MH, Roniker B, Krause SL, et al. (2002). Eplerenone, a selective aldosterone blocker, in mild-to-moderate hypertension. *American Journal of Hypertension;* 15: 709–16.

Wright JT Jr, Dunn JK, Cutler JA, et al. (2005). Outcomes in hypertensive black and nonblack patients treated with chlortalidone, amlodipine, and lisinopril. *Journal of American Medical Association;* 293: 1595–608.

Chapter 13

Beta blockers in hypertension

Sunil Nadar

Key points

- Beta blockers act by blocking the beta-adrenergic receptors in the body.
- At one time, they were the first-line monotherapeutic agents for the treatment of hypertension.
- Recent trial data suggest that they are not as effective as other agents in lowering blood pressure and in reducing the risk of cardiovascular and cerebrovascular events.
- Current guidelines recommend that they be used only in case of compelling indications such as acute coronary syndromes, ischaemic heart disease, and heart failure.

13.1 Types of beta blockers

Beta blockers can be classified based on their receptor selectivity, intrinsic sympathomimetic activity (ISA), associated alpha blockade, and other properties like peripheral vasodilatation (nebivolol). A list of beta blockers based on these properties is illustrated in Table 13.1.

13.2 Mechanism of action

Beta blockers block the action of endogenous catecholamines (adrenaline and noradrenaline) on the beta-adrenergic receptors. There are three known types of beta receptors designated beta-1, beta-2, and beta-3. Beta-1 adrenergic receptors are located mainly in the heart and the kidneys. Beta-2 adrenergic receptors are located mainly in the lungs, gastrointestinal tract, liver, vascular smooth muscle, uterus, and skeletal muscles, whereas beta-3 adrenergic receptors are located in the fat cells.

Effects of beta-1 receptor blockade on the heart include a negative chronotropic and ionotropic effect causing decreased cardiac conduction velocity and automaticity. Stimulation of beta-1 receptors in kidneys causes renin release. Beta blockers therefore should reduce plasma renin levels in patients with hypertension. Although a primary association between the antihypertensive effect of beta blockers and plasma renin activity is not established, a significant reduction in blood pressure is noted in patients with high pre-treatment renin levels when treated with a beta blocker. Stimulation of beta-2 receptors induces smooth muscle relaxation resulting in vasodilatation and brochodilatation. Beta blockers were initially contraindicated in hypertension as it was thought that this beta-2 receptor blockade would lead to vasoconstriction and worsening of hypertension. However, subsequent studies disproved this and in fact showed that patients receiving propranolol in a varying dose of 30–400 mg a day had an average fall of 19/7 mmHg in supine blood pressure.

Table 13.1 Various beta blockers and their properties

Drug	B1 selectivity	ISA activity	Lipid solubility	Alpha blockade
Acebutolol	+	+	+	−
Atenolol	++	−	−	−
Betaxolol	++	−	−	−
Bisoprolol	+++	−	+	−
Bucindolol	−	−	+	−
Carteolol	−	+	−	−
Carvedilol	−	−	+++	+
Celiprolol	++	+	−	−
Esmolol	++	−	−	−
Labetalol	−	−	++	+
Metoprolol	++	−	++	−
Nebivolol	++	−	++	−
Penbutolol	−	+	+++	−
Pindolol	−	+++	++	−

The antihypertensive mechanism appears to involve the following:

• Reduction in cardiac output (due to negative chronotropic and ionotropic effects),

• Reduction in renin release from the kidneys, and

• Effect on the central nervous system to reduce sympathetic activity.

13.3 **Role of beta blockers in hypertension**

Various studies have shown that beta blockers are effective in reducing blood pressure when compared to placebo; however, there are no studies to prove that their monotherapeutic use in hypertension leads to reduced mortality and morbidity when compared to placebo. Role of beta blockers in hypertension needs to be discussed in patients with or without any associated compelling indications such as ischemic heart disease, heart failure, diabetes, chronic kidney disease, cerebrovascular disease, elderly and ethnic minorities, etc.

Despite paucity or even absence of data showing beneficial effects of beta blockers, these drugs and diuretics were considered to be the first-line of antihypertensive therapy from 1983 to 1997. More recent guidelines (see Chapter 21) do not recommend beta blockers as first-line monotherapy because, as discussed below, beta blockers are not as effective as the other agents in lowering blood pressure and in preventing cardiovascular and cerebrovascular endpoints.

Clinical trials show that beta blockers are less potent than other agents in lowering blood pressure. Blood pressure control was achieved in less than 50% of patients randomized to the atenolol arm in the Losartan Intervention For Endpoint reduction in hypertension (LIFE) trial and less than 10% of the patients remained on monotherapy of beta blockers. In the first Swedish Trial in Old Patients with hypertension (STOP 1) trial, blood pressure control was half as effective when treated with beta blockers as compared with diuretics. In the ASCOT-BPLA study, patients treated with amlodipine-based treatment resulted in 1.7 mmHg mean lower systolic and 2.0 mmHg lower diastolic blood pressure as compared to atenolol-based treatment. This was associated with a 23% lower risk of stroke and 14% lower risk of coronary events for the amlodipine arm as compared to the atenolol arm.

In the Medical Research Council (MRC) study, treatment with a diuretic was associated with a lower risk of cardiovascular events compared with that with the beta blocker, even after adjusting for the decrease in blood pressure. This allows the speculation that either the diuretic confers a specific benefit irrespective of the decrease in arterial pressure or, more concerning, that the beta blocker confers an ill effect on the cardiovascular system in the elderly that overrides the beneficial effect of a decrease in arterial pressure.

Messereli and colleagues (1998) assessed the antihypertensive efficacy of beta blockers as compared to diuretics in a systematic analysis of ten randomized trials in elderly patients. Their results showed that two-thirds of patients treated with diuretics were well controlled on monotherapy as compared to less than a third of patients who had well-controlled blood pressure when treated with beta-blocker monotherapy. Their analysis also suggested that diuretics were superior to beta-blocker therapy with regards to preventing cerebrovascular events, fatal stroke, and cardiovascular and all-cause mortality. Beta blockers reduce the risk of stroke by 16–22% when compared with placebo. This risk reduction is lower than the 38% reduction for the same degree of blood pressure reduction observed with the use of other antihypertensive agents. Furthermore, beta blockers provide no benefit for the end points of all-cause mortality, cardiovascular mortality, and myocardial infarction when compared with other antihypertensive agents. Other meta-analyses have shown that there is a 24% and 30% greater risk of stroke with the use of beta blockers when compared with CCBs and blockers of the renin–angiotensin–aldosterone system (RAAS) respectively, with the risk being greater in elderly patients as compared to that in younger patients (Tables 13.2–13.3).

Beta blockers have been shown to be less effective in controlling the central aortic pressure as compared to the peripheral brachial blood pressure measurements. In the Conduit Artery Functional Endpoint (CAFE) study, for the same peripheral arterial blood pressure, atenolol-/bendroflumethizide-based treatment resulted in a 4.3 mmHg greater central aortic systolic blood pressure and a 3 mmHg greater central aortic pulse pressure as compared with amlodipine-/perindopril-based treatment.

A recent Cochrane review by Wiysonge and colleagues demonstrated that beta blockers are inferior to various CCBs for all-cause mortality, stroke, and total cardiovascular events, and to

Table 13.2 Overview of major meta-analyses of randomized controlled trials of beta blockers in patients with hypertension versus placebo				
Meta-analysis	No. of trials	Mortality	Myocardial infarction	Stroke
Cochrane 2007	4	0.99 (0.88–1.11)	0.93 (0.81–1.07)	0.80 (0.66–0.96)
Bradley et al. 2006	4	0.99 (0.88–1.11)	0.93 (0.81–1.07)	0.80 (0.66–0.96)
Khan et al. 2006	5	0.91 (0.74–1.12)	0.98 (0.83–1.16)	0.78 (0.63–0.98)
Lindholm et al. 2005	7	0.95 (0.86–1.04)	0.93 (0.83–1.05)	0.81 (0.71–0.93)
Carlberg et al. 2004 (atenolol)	4	1.01 (0.89–1.15)	0.99 (0.83–1.19)	0.85 (0.72–1.01)
Numbers represent hazard ratio (HR) (95% confidence interval).				

Table 13.3 Overview of major meta-analyses of randomized controlled trials of beta blockers in patients with hypertension versus other antihypertensive agents

Meta-analysis	No. of trials	Mortality	Myocardial infarction	Stroke
Khan *et al.* 2006	5	0.97 (0.83–1.14)	0.97 (0.86–1.10)	0.99 (0.67–1.44)
Khan *et al.* 2006	7	1.05 (0.99–1.11)	1.06 (0.94–1.20)	1.18 (1.07–1.30)
Lindholm *et al.* 2005	13	1.03 (0.99–1.08)	1.02 (0.93–1.12)	1.16 (1.04–1.30)
Carlberg *et al.* 2004 (atenolol)	5	1.13 (0.97–1.33)	1.04 (0.89–1.20)	1.30 (1.12–1.50)

Numbers represent hazard ratio (95% confidence interval).

renin–angiotensin system inhibition for stroke. Similar findings were obtained in meta-analysis of the role of beta blockers by Lindholm and colleagues. In another meta-analysis, Khan and McAlister found beta blockers to be inferior to all other therapies in effects on both a composite outcome of major cardiovascular events (stroke, myocardial infarction, and death) and stroke for elderly hypertensive patients but found no difference in effects for younger patients. All these authors conclude that the available evidence does not support the use of beta blockers as first-line drugs in the treatment of hypertension.

Of interest, the recent guidelines issued by the European Society of Hypertension and the European Society of Cardiology are not so negative about the use of beta blockers. They recommend that beta blockers can still be used as a first-line antihypertensive agent as they have considerable benefit in patients with a recent heart attack or those with heart failure. However, they do mention that given their propensity to increase weight and cause unfavourable metabolic changes, they are best avoided in patients with multiple cardiovascular risk factors, including the metabolic syndrome and its major components—that is, abdominal obesity, high normal or impaired fasting glucose, and impaired glucose tolerance, conditions that make the risk of incident diabetes higher.

13.4 **Beta blockers and ischaemic heart disease**

Ischaemic heart disease is the most common form of target organ damage associated with hypertension. In patients with hypertension and stable angina pectoris, the first drug of choice is usually a beta blocker. In patients with stable angina and no prior myocardial infarction it has been suggested that CCBs may be beneficial, as they do not have the adverse effects of beta blockers on insulin resistance, weight gain, decreased exercise tolerance, and sexual dysfunction.

There is good evidence that beta blockers reduce mortality in patients with prior myocardial infarction. Analyses from prospective randomized trials suggest that beta blockers reduce mortality by 23% and reduce mortality by up to 40% in observational studies. Treatment of 84 patients for a period of one year prevents one death and treatment of 107 patients for a year prevents one episode of non-fatal reinfarction. The numbers needed to treat to achieve mortality reduction is far fewer with beta blockers as compared to antiplatelet agents and statins.

In patients with acute coronary syndromes, early treatment with intravenous beta blockers has shown mixed results. The TIMI-2B (Thrombolysis In Myocardial Infraction) study, ISIS-1(International study of Infarct Survival) study, and the MIAMI (Metoprolol In Acute

Myocardial Infarction) study showed favourable effects of early initiation of intravenous beta blockade, whereas the GUSTO (Global Utilization of Streptokinase and Tissue plasminogen Activator for Occluded Coronary Arteries) trial showed that early beta blockage resulted in 30% increased risk of death along with a greater incidence of heart failure, shock, and pacemaker use.

13.5 **Heart failure and beta blockers**

Beta blockers were initially considered contraindicated in heart failure because of initial negative ionotropic effects. However, there have been large studies such as the CIBIS-II (The Cardiac Insufficiency Bisoprolol Study II) and the MERIT-HF (Metoprolol Randomized Intervention Trial in congestive heart failure) study in chronic heart failure demonstrating significant improvement in mortality and morbidity with the use of beta-blocker therapy in patients with heart failure secondary to left ventricular systolic dysfunction. Multiple meta-analyses have shown benefit of beta-blocker therapy in patients with heart failure irrespective of their gender, age, and presence or absence of diabetes.

In diastolic heart failure, beta blockers may be used to decrease heart rate (dromotropic effects) and thereby increase the duration of diastole, which can potentially improve the haemodynamic response to exercise. There is limited evidence that propranolol treatment can reduce mortality and LV mass in patients with heart failure symptoms and a previous history of myocardial infarction, but preserved LV systolic function. However, there is no significant improvement in radionuclide parameters of LV diastolic relaxation in a study of patients with moderate systolic heart failure when treated with either carvedilol or placebo. Using echocardiographic parameters, Pallazuoli and colleagues (2004) suggest that carvedilol therapy does modify diastolic filling favourably—the restrictive transmitral Doppler filling pattern was seen to change back towards a 'pseudonormal' pattern following carvedilol treatment. Larger-scale investigations would be necessary to confirm these findings.

13.6 **Beta blockers and diabetes**

Beta blockers have been shown to increase insulin resistance and predispose to diabetes. In a meta-analysis of 22 clinical trials, the risk of diabetes with beta blockers and diuretics was much higher than with placebo. In another large meta-analysis of 12 studies evaluating 94 492 patients, beta-blocker therapy resulted in a 22% increased risk for new-onset diabetes compared to non-diuretic antihypertensive agents. A higher baseline body mass index and higher baseline fasting glucose levels were a significant predictor of new-onset diabetes mellitus. The risk for diabetes was greater with atenolol, and in the elderly.

Possible mechanism leading to development of diabetes include weight gain, attenuation of beta-receptor-mediated release of insulin from the pancreatic beta cells, and decreased blood flow in the skeletal muscle tissue leading to decreased insulin sensitivity. Beta blockers can also produce hypoglycaemic unawareness because of their autonomic blockade.

In the Glycaemic Effects in Diabetes Mellitus Carvedilol-Metoprolol Comparison in Hypertensives (GEMINI) trial there was an increase in the HBA1c on treatment with metoprolol but not with carvedilol, suggesting that all beta blockers may not have similar effects on diabetes.

13.7 **Beta blockers effect on left ventricular hypertrophy**

Left ventricular hypertrophy remains a strong predictor of cardio-vascular mortality and morbidity and its regression lowers the risk irrespective of blood pressure reduction. In a meta-analysis on the effects of various antihypertensive therapies on LVH regression, beta blockers were found to be inferior to diuretics, calcium antagonists, ACE inhibitors, and ARBs. In the LIFE study, therapy with losartan resulted in greater LVH regression as compared to therapy with atenolol for almost similar blood pressure reductions.

13.8 **Beta blockers and weight gain**

Use of beta-blocker therapy has been associated with a small but systematic weight gain. Only a minority of clinical trials with beta blockers report weight changes during treatment. In trials that do report weight changes, beta blockers are associated with a weight gain of 1.2 kg (range 0.4–3.5). This may be attributed to the fact that beta blockade can decrease metabolic rate and also have other negative effects on energy metabolism. Obesity management in overweight hypertensive patients may therefore be more difficult in the presence of beta-blocker treatment.

13.9 **Beta blockers in black patients**

The prevalence, severity, and impact of hypertension are increased in black patients, who also demonstrate somewhat reduced blood pressure responses to monotherapy with beta blockers, ACE inhibitors, or ARBs compared with diuretics or CCBs. In black patients, efficacy of beta blockers in reducing systolic blood pressure is no different as compared to placebo and there are reports that beta blockers may even increase systolic blood pressure in these patients.

Therefore, when beta-blocker therapy is not effective in reducing blood pressure, clinicians should discontinue therapy rather than increasing the drug dose.

13.10 **Beta blockers in pregnant women**

Beta blockers have been used during pregnancy to treat hypertension and thyrotoxicosis, and for rate control of atrial fibrillation. Pharmacodynamics of beta blockers in pregnant women is relatively well-studied, and serious maternal side effects are rare. Foetal pharmacodynamic and foetal side effects are less well known, and reports in the literature are sometimes contradictory. The safety of these agents, particularly atenolol and propranolol, is somewhat controversial because of individual reports of adverse effects on the foetus.

A meta-analysis of 13 trials (1480 women) comparing beta blockers with placebo or no beta blocker showed that beta-blocker therapy decreased the risk of severe hypertension and the need for additional antihypertensives. There was insufficient data for conclusions about the effect on perinatal mortality or preterm birth. Beta blockers also seemed to be associated with an increase in small-for-gestational-age (SGA) infants. Eleven trials have compared beta-blocker therapy with methyldopa. Beta blockers appear to be no more effective and probably equally safe. Labetalol, a beta blocker that also has alpha-blocking properties, is a common second-line agent that is used.

13.11 **Beta blockers and their effect on quality of life**

The possible effects of beta blockers on various aspects of quality of life have been long debated, including an adverse impact on normal exercise capacity, cognitive function, sleep quality, overall mood, and sexual function (erectile failure in men and depressed libido in both sexes). Furthermore, there have been studies reporting impairment of memory function, particularly with the use of non-selective agents such as propranolol. The lipophilic forms of beta blockers (such as propranolol) can cause cognitive impairment during diurnal activity and in addition, inhibit REM sleep and sleep quality.

Large-scale epidemiological studies also suggest a link between an increased use of antidepressant medications within 12 months of the prescription of a beta blocker, as compared to a reference group of patients treated for chronic diseases. However, such associations are frequently confounded and in one double blind, randomized, controlled cross-over study there appears to be no significant effect on cognitive function. Indeed, one placebo-controlled trial in 312 hypertensive patients suggested that propranolol causes no greater impairment of cognitive function than placebo.

Beta-blocker therapy could be implicated in sexual dysfunction, both by vasodilator effects on male erection and more generally by decreased libido. There have been several cross-over studies reporting reduction of sexual activity in hypertensive men on treatment with beta blockers compared to active controls such as lisinopril or valsartan. Unfortunately, these frequently do not define the mechanical or psychosexual nature of the dysfunction. While there are many mechanistic hypotheses such as reductions in the levels of testosterone in males receiving beta blockers as compared to other antihypertensive medications, these studies are far from definitive and always fail to show relevance to practical sexual/erectile function assessment.

13.12 **Third-generation beta blockers**

Third-generation beta blockers are distinguished from the earlier class of beta blockers by their vasodilating activity and show more promise in their clinical effects. Nebivolol is a third-generation lipophilic beta blocker with distinct beta-1 selective and vasodilating properties. A number of experimental and human studies suggest that nebivolol increases the bioavailability of nitric oxide (NO) and this results in vasodilatation and improved endothelial function. It also appears to have antioxidant properties, and studies have shown that it causes greater central aortic pressure reductions than atenolol in human subjects. The pharmocological profile is characterized by the significant antihypertensive effect as well as lowering of cardiac preload and afterload. These effects suggest that nebivolol may be beneficial in heart failure patients as well. The randomized trial to determine the effect of nebivolol on mortality and cardiovascular hospital admission in elderly patients with heart failure (SENIORS) has demonstrated that it is effective and well tolerated in elderly patients with heart failure. In general, nebivolol is well tolerated and does not appear to significantly influence glucose or plasma lipid metabolism and this also is a major breakthrough in comparison with the older beta blockers. It is also devoid of any ISA.

13.13 **Contraindications**

The absolute contraindications for the use of beta blockers include severe asthma, and obstructive airways disease as these agents can cause bronchospasm, heart blocks and bradyarrhythmias, and hypotension and shock.

They should be used with caution in severe decompensated heart failure, in peripheral vascular disease and in patients with poorly controlled insulin dependent diabetes. They should also be used cautiously in patients suspected to have a phaeochromocytoma as unopposed alpha-adrenergic agonist action may lead to a serious hypertensive crisis.

Key references

Bangalore S, Messerli FH, Kostis JB, *et al.* (2007). Cardiovascular protection using beta-blockers: a critical review of the evidence. *Journal of the American College of Cardiology*; 50(7): 563–72.

Bradley HA, Wiysonge CS, Volmink JA, *et al.* (2006). How strong is the evidence for use of beta-blockers as first-line therapy for hypertension? Systematic review and meta-analysis. *Journal of Hypertension*; 24(11): 2131–41.

Brewster LM, van Montfrans GA, Kleijnen J (2004). Systematic review: antihypertensive drug therapy in black patients. *Annals of Internal Medicines*; 141(8): 614–27.

Carlberg B, Samuelsson O, Lindholm LH (2004). Atenolol in hypertension: is it a wise choice? *Lancet*; 364(9446): 1684–9.

Larochelle P, Tobe SV, Lacourciere Y (2014). Beta blockers in hypertension: studies and meta-analyses over the years. *Canadian Journal of Cardiology*; 30(5 suppl): S16–22.

Lindholm LH, Carlberg B, Samuelsson O (2005). Should beta blockers remain first choice in treatment of primary hypertension? A meta-analysis. *Lancet*; 366: 1545–53.

Messerli FH, Grossman E, Goldbourt U (1998). Are beta-blockers efficacious as first-line therapy for hypertension in the elderly? A systematic review. *Journal of American Medical Association*; 279(23): 1903–7.

Wiysonge CS, Bradley H, Volmink J, *et al.* (2012). Beta-blockers for hypertension. *Cochrane Database of Systematic Reviews*; 15; 8: CD002003.

Chapter 14

Calcium-channel blockers and hypertension

Sunil Nadar

> ### Key points
>
> - Calcium-channel blockers are a diverse group of drugs that are very effective in lowering blood pressure.
> - Clinical trials have shown that their use results in improved cardiovascular outcomes in patients at high cardiovascular risk.
> - Current guidelines recommend that these agents be used as first-line drugs in the treatment of hypertension.
> - They are generally well tolerated.

14.1 Introduction

Calcium-channel blockers have been a useful tool in the management of hypertension for many years. The term was first used by Fleckenstein in 1969 to describe a compound which was both negatively inotropic and a coronary vasodilator. Verapamil was one of the very first calcium-channel blockers introduced but since then there have been several other agents with similar pharmacological modes of action. Unlike beta-adrenoceptor blockers, however, calcium-channel blockers do not share a common molecular structure.

14.2 Mechanism of action

Calcium entry into cells activates the contractile system in the smooth muscle and cardiac fibre. Conversely, reduction in the amount of intracellular calcium reduces myocardial contractility as well as inducing peripheral and coronary vasodilatation. Although all calcium-channel blockers by their very nature share the common property of inhibiting cellular calcium influx, they possess differing effects on vascular smooth muscle, cardiac myocytes, and the cardiac conductive tissue. Essentially, a calcium-channel blocker acts by inhibiting the cellular entry of calcium through voltage-dependent L- and T-type calcium channels. Despite sharing a common mechanism of action, the available agents possess differing molecular structure and site of binding. Three classes of agents have been identified: dihydropyridines (nifedipine and amlodipine), benzothiazepine (diltiazem), and phenylalkylamine (verapamil). Calcium-channel blockers thus possess chemical and pharmacological heterogeneity and are capable of blocking calcium channels in differing locations with varying degrees of intensity. For example, phenylalkylamines, such as verapamil, have a greater degree of affinity for cardiac conduction tissue, whereas others such as dihydropyridines (nifedipine and amlodipine) act on the smooth muscle cells of the resistance vessels. Benzothiazepines such as diltiazem have proportionate action on both the heart and smooth muscle cells of resistance vessels.

Although all three subclasses of calcium-channel blockers have been widely used, second-generation dihydropyridines (amlodipine, nifedipine, and felodipine) and heart-rate reducing non-dihydropyridines such as verapamil are the ones most often used as antihypertensive agents. Basic subclasses and molecular structures of the commonly used calcium-channel blockers are summarized in Figure 14.1.

14.3 **Clinical evidence for the use of calcium blockers in hypertension**

Several randomized clinical trials have demonstrated the efficacy of calcium-channel blockers in the management of hypertension. The largest of these trials is the ALLHAT (Antihypertensive and Lipid Lowering to prevent Heart Attack Trial). This prospective, randomized controlled study recruited 33 357 hypertensive subjects who had one additional cardiovascular risk factor to one of four agents: chlortalidone, lisinopril, amlodipine, or doxazosin. Aside from the doxazosin arm, which was terminated early because of an excess of admissions for heart failure, remaining treatment arms were followed up for a mean of 4.9 years. At follow-up there was no significant difference noted between three treatment arms for the primary outcome (fatal or non-fatal myocardial infarction). Mean blood pressure reduction in the amlodipine-treated group was 11.5 ± 9.3 mmHg with 40% of patients requiring an additional agent(s) as per study protocol. Systolic blood pressure reduction was greater with chlortalidone compared with lisinopril or amlodipine.

Another large randomized controlled trial, VALUE (Valsartan Antihypertensive Long-term Use Evaluation Trial), compared amlodipine to valsartan in 15 245 patients with hypertension and multiple cardiovascular risk factors (previously treated with two or more medications) and demonstrated the superiority of amlodipine to valsartan in blood pressure reduction. Amlodipine was shown to lower blood pressure by 17.3 ± 9.9 mmHg compared to 15.2 ± 8.2 mmHg in the valsartan group. The antihypertensive effect of amlodipine was greatest in the first six months of the trial, and this was associated with a lower event rate within this time period. The final endpoint, however, showed no differences in event rates between both treatment arms.

The CONVINCE study (Controlled ONset Verapamil INvestigation of Cardiovascular Endpoints) examined the head-to-head efficacy of calcium-channel blockers to beta blockers. A total of 16 602 hypertensive patients with one additional risk factor were randomized to receive either controlled-onset extended-release (COER) verapamil or atenolol with the addition of a diuretic as second-line agent if required. There was no significant difference in blood pressure reduction between the two treatment groups (13.6 ± 7.8 mmHg for verapamil compared to 13.5 ± 7.1 mmHg in the beta blocker group). In addition, there was no observed difference in the primary outcome of cardiovascular-related death between treatment groups.

The INVEST (International Verapamil Trandolapril Study) examined 22 576 patients with hypertension and established coronary artery disease. Patients were randomized to either sustained release verapamil with trandolapril and hydrochlorothiazide as stepped regimens, or twice daily atenolol plus daily hydrochlorothiazide and trandolapril as stepped regimens. Mean blood pressure reduction was similar in both groups with no difference in the primary outcome (all-cause mortality, non-fatal myocardial infarction, or non-fatal stroke).

The ASCOT-BPLA study (Anglo Scandinavian Cardiovascular Outcomes Trial–Blood Pressure Lowering Arm) compared amlodipine with atenolol for the prevention of coronary heart disease in 19 342 hypertensive patients with no previous documented coronary disease. The study was stopped prematurely after 5.5 years after observing a significant benefit of using a calcium antagonist on the primary endpoint. Amlodipine use was associated with less stroke,

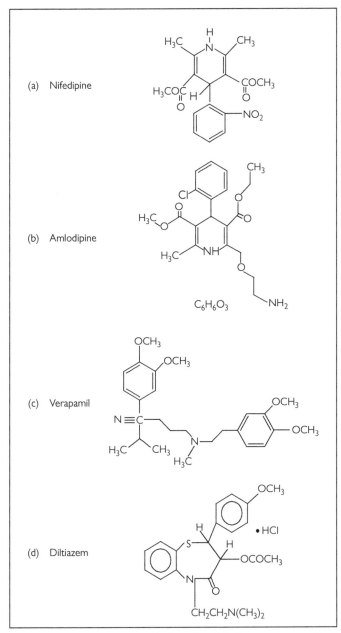

Figure 14.1 Classes and molecular structure of calcium-channel blockers in current use: (a) nifedipine, (b) amlodipine, (c) verapamil, and (d) diltiazem

Table 14.1 Summary of trial evidence demonstrating the efficacy of calcium-channel blockers as antihypertensive agents

Trial	Trial subjects	Findings
ALLHAT (Antihypertensive and Lipid Lowering to prevent Heart Attack Trial)	33 357 hypertensives with one additional risk factor	Amlodipine equivalent to other agents in reducing myocardial infarction
VALUE (Valsartan Antihypertensive Long-term Use Evaluation Trial)	15 245 hypertensives with multiple additional risk factors	Amlodipine superior to valsartan in blood pressure reduction. No difference in cardio-vascular event rate
CONVINCE study (Controlled ONset Verapamil INvestigation of Cardiovascular Endpoints)	16 602 hypertensives with one additional risk factor	Verapamil equivalent to atenolol in blood pressure reduction and cardiovascular outcome
INVEST (International Verapamil Trandolapril Study)	22 576 hypertensives with coronary disease	Verapamil provides equivalent blood pressure reduction to trandolapril and no difference in total and cardiovascular mortality
ASCOT–BPLA study (Anglo Scandinavian Cardiovascular Outcomes Trial–Blood Pressure Lowering Arm)	19 342 hypertensives with no previous coronary disease	Amlodipine demonstrates superior reduction in total and cardiovascular mortality and also reduces the incidence of developing diabetes
NORDIL study (NORdic DILtiazem)	10 881 patients with diastolic blood pressure > 100 mmHg	Diltiazem equivalent to other agents in reducing all-cause and cardiovascular mortality
INSIGHT study (International Nifedipine GITS Study of Intervention as a Goal in Hypertension Treatment)	6321 hypertensives with one additional risk factor	Nifedipine equivalent to co-amilozide in reducing cardiovascular mortality

total cardiovascular events, and all-cause mortality. In addition, there was a lower incidence of developing diabetes in the amlodipine-treated group.

Evidence for diltiazem use as an antihypertensive agent comes from the NORDIL study (NORdic DILtiazem). This was a prospective, randomized, open, blinded endpoint study, enrolling 10 881 patients, aged 50–74 years, at health centres in Norway and Sweden, who had diastolic blood pressure of 100 mmHg or more. Patients were randomly assigned diltiazem, or diuretics, beta blockers, or both. Diltiazem was found to be as effective as treatment based on diuretics, beta blockers, or both in preventing the combined primary endpoint of all stroke, myocardial infarction, and other cardiovascular death. Systolic blood pressure reduction was slightly greater in the combined diuretic/beta-blocker group compared to the diltiazem group.

The INSIGHT study (International Nifedipine GITS Study of Intervention as a Goal in Hypertension Treatment) compared the effects of the calcium-channel blocker nifedipine once daily with the diuretic combination co-amilozide on cardiovascular mortality and morbidity in high-risk patients with hypertension. This was a prospective, randomized, double-blind trial in Europe and Israel in 6321 patients aged 55–80 years with hypertension (blood pressure ≥ 150/95 mmHg, or ≥ 160 mmHg systolic). Patients also had at least one additional cardiovascular risk factor. Nifedipine once daily and co-amilozide were equally effective in preventing overall cardiovascular or cerebrovascular complications.

There is therefore a large body of clinical evidence to support the efficacy of calcium-channel blockers in the treatment of hypertension. The clinical trials suggest that these agents are both efficacious in cardiovascular event prevention and in blood pressure reduction compared to other agents. Table 14.1 is a summary of the main clinical trials involving calcium-channel blockers in hypertension.

14.4 Use of calcium-channel blockers in proteinuric nephropathy

Calcium-channel antagonist groups also have a divergent role in reno-protection. In hypertensive patients with proteinuria (> 300 mg protein per gram of creatinine) use of dihydropyridine calcium-channel blockers have failed to slow the progression of nephropathy and if used as antihypertensive agents, they must be used in conjunction with ACE inhibitors or angiotensin II receptor antagonists. In contrast, a systematic review of 28 clinical trials by Bakris and colleagues (2004) suggested that while dihydropyridine and non-dihydropyridine calcium blockers were similarly efficacious at reducing blood pressure, non-dihyrdropyridine calcium blockers demonstrate greater reductions in proteinuria in patients with nephropathy (with or without diabetes).

14.5 Adverse events, safety, and tolerability of calcium-channel blockers

Typical adverse effects experienced by patients taking calcium-channel blockers in the first few weeks of therapy include flushing, peripheral oedema, hypotension, tachycardia, rash, headache, and constipation. The list is not exhaustive but often these initial adverse effects disappear after a few weeks of treatment.

The use of calcium-channel blockers in hypertension has not been without controversy. Initially, an increase in the incidence of acute myocardial infarction was noted in trials of nifedipine. An initial meta-analysis then highlighted these drugs as potentially dangerous in their long-term use—examining 27 743 patients in nine clinical trials, suggesting an increase risk of myocardial infarction, heart failure, and major cardiovascular events. A contradictory analysis from the Blood Pressure Lowering Treatments Trialists' Collaboration did not find any increased risk in the use of calcium-channel blockers. Further supportive evidence for the safety and efficacy of calcium blockers has been reported in three more recent meta-analyses: a further two reports from the Blood Pressure Lowering Treatments Trialists' Collaboration both examining 27 trials (136 124 patients in one and 158 709 patients including 33 395 with diabetes in the other), and Staesson and colleagues (2002) looking at nine trials (65 605 patients). These meta-analyses supported the efficacy of calcium blockers in the reduction and prevention of major cardiovascular events and showed no evidence of increased incidence of heart failure. The increased incidence of fatal myocardial infarction was noted only in one trial (INSIGHT).

In terms of heart failure prevention, dihydropyridine calcium-channel blockers have a neutral effect on mortality and hospitalizations in systolic heart failure. However, verapamil and diltiazem have negative inotropic effects and should not be utilized in patients demonstrating left ventricular systolic impairment.

The other major contraindications to their use are the presence of cardiac conduction abnormalities (for the non-dihydropyridines).

14.6 Summary and recommendations

Calcium-channel blockers are effective antihypertensive agents and multiple clinical trial evidence points to their efficacy in treating hypertension, either as a single agent or in conjunction with other antihypertensives. The recent British Hypertension Society guidelines and European guidelines (2013) recommend that they are used as first-line agents in patients above the age of 55 and those of African or Carribbean descent. Thiazides are also a first-line alternative agent for this group. Calcium-channel blockers are also recommended as first line in isolated systolic hypertension, patients with LVH and women. They have been shown to reduce long-term cardiovascular risk and are generally well tolerated. They should not be used in patients with left ventricular systolic impairment, and only non-dihydropyridine calcium-channel blockers should be considered for use in proteinuric nephropathy, preferable in conjunction with an agent that blocks the renin–angiotensin–aldosterone system. Nifedipine is the only calcium antagonist that has been safely tested for use in pregnancy.

Along with ACE inhibitors, calcium-channel blockers are also recommended for use in diabetics and patients with metabolic syndrome (which is considered pre-diabetic). Meta-analyses also suggest that calcium antagonists have a slightly higher efficacy in stroke prevention and in delaying the progression of carotid atherosclerosis than diuretics and beta blockers.

Key references

Bakris GL, Weir MR, Secic M, et al. (2004). Differential effects of calcium antagonist subclasses on markers of nephropathy progression. *Kidney International;*, 65 (6): 1991–2002.

Costanzo P, Perrone-Filardi P, Petretta M, et al. (2009). Calcium channel blockers and cardiovascular outcomes: a meta-analysis of 175,634 patients. *Journal of Hypertension;* 27: 1136–51.

Dahlöf B, Sever PS, Poulter NR, et al. ASCOT Investigators. (2005). Prevention of cardiovascular events with an antihypertensive regimen of amlodipine adding perindopril as required versus atenolol adding bendroflumethiazide as required, in the Anglo-Scandinavian Cardiac Outcomes Trial-Blood Pressure Lowering Arm (ASCOT-BPLA): a multicentre randomised controlled trial. *Lancet;* 366(9489): 895–906.

Julius S, Kjeldsen SE, Weber M, et al. (2004). Outcomes in hypertensive patients at high cardiovascular risk treated with regimens based on valsartan or amlodipine: the VALUE randomised trial. *Lancet;* 363(9426): 2022–31.

ALLHAT Collaborative Research Group (2004). Major cardiovascular events in hypertensive patients randomized to doxazosin vs chlortalidone: the antihypertensive and lipid-lowering treatment to prevent heart attack trial (ALLHAT). *Journal of American Medical Association;* 283(15): 1967–75.

Nathan S, Pepine CJ, Bakris GL, et al. (2005). Calcium antagonists. Effects on cardiorenal risk in hypertensive patients. *Hypertension;* 46: 637–42.

Neal B, MacMahon S, Chapman N. Blood Pressure Lowering Treatment Trialists' Collaboration. (2000). Effects of ACE inhibitors, calcium antagonists, and other blood-pressure-lowering drugs: results of prospectively designed overviews of randomised trials. *Lancet;* 356 (9246): 1955–64.

Pahor M, Psaty BM, Alderman MH (2000). Health outcomes associated with calcium antagonists compared with other first-line antihypertensive therapies: a meta-analysis of randomised controlled trials. *Lancet;* 356(9246): 1949–54.

Rothwell PM, Howard SC, Dolan E, et al. (2010) Effects of beta blockers and calcium-channel blockers on within-individual variability in blood pressure and risk of stroke. *Lancet Neurology;* 9: 469–80.

Singh BN (1986). The mechanisms of action of calcium antagonists relative to their clinical application. *British Journal of Clinical Pharmacology;* 21 (Suppl 2): 109–22.

Staessen JA, Wang JG, Thijs L (2002). Calcium-channel blockade and cardiovascular prognosis: recent evidence from clinical outcome trials. *American Journal of Hypertension;* 15(7 Pt 2): 85S–93S.

The Task Force for the management of arterial hypertension of the European Society of Hypertension (ESH) and of the European Society of Cardiology (2013). ESH/ESC Guidelines for the management of arterial hypertension *European Heart Journal;* 34, 2159–19.

Chapter 15

ACE inhibitors in hypertension

Sunil Nadar

Key points

- Angiotensin-converting enzyme (ACE) inhibitors decrease the production of angiotensin II, reduce sympathetic nervous system activity, and increase bradykinin levels.
- ACE inhibitors are effective antihypertensive agents and slow the progression of target organ damage including various nephropathies and left ventricular hypertrophy and heart failure.
- They are also useful in reducing the mortality post-myocardial infarction and in high-risk coronary or peripheral vascular disease patients.
- The main side effects of ACE inhibitors include cough, angioedema, hyperkalaemia, and worsening of renal functions especially in the presence of renal artery stenosis.

15.1 Introduction

The renin–angiotensin–aldosterone system (RAAS) plays an important role in the pathophysiology of hypertension as it affects the vascular tone, regulation of fluid volume, electrolyte balance, and blood volume.

Renin is synthesized and secreted from the renal juxta glomerular cells located in the walls of afferent arterioles which are contiguous with macula densa. Renin converts angiotensinogen (which is a protein synthesized in the liver) to angiotensin I (a decapeptide). The angiotensin I which is inert is converted to angiotensin II, an octapeptide, by angiotensin-converting enzyme (ACE) which is present in the pulmonary circulation and vascular endothelium. Angiotensin II is the active form and it leads to vasoconstriction and salt retention (via aldosterone release).

It had been apparent since the 1970s that targeting the RAAS would help reduce blood pressure. Inhibitors of the ACE or ACE inhibitors (ACEI) were the first substances produced to target the RAAS. They were introduced first in 1977 and now with the clinical evidence that is available regarding their use in hypertension, they are one of the mainstays in the management of hypertension.

15.2 Pharmacology

15.2.1 Pharmacokinetics

The pharmacological actions of the different agents belonging to this group are summarized in Table 15.1. With the exception of lisinopril and captopril, they are prodrugs that improve absorption but require hydrolysis prior to having any biological effect. In general, these drugs are well absorbed orally and generally have a short half-life, with the exception of perindopril.

Drug	Prodrug	Half-life (hours)	Route of elimination	Dose (mg) per day	Time to maximum effect (hours)
Captopril	No	2	Renal	25–150	1
Fosinopril	Yes	12	Renal and hepatic	10–40	46
Enalapril	Yes	11	Renal	5–40	46
Trandolapril	Yes	16–24	Renal and hepatic	1–4	68
Quinapril	Yes	3	Renal	10–80	4
Perindopril	Yes	9	Renal	4–8	34
Lisinopril	No	13	Renal	5–40	46
Ramipril	Yes	12	Renal and hepatic	1.25–10	36
Benazepril	Yes	21	Renal and hepatic	5–40	24

Table 15.1 Characteristics of the various drugs in this class

They are mainly eliminated via the kidneys, although some are excreted via the liver. These drugs vary by the type of side-chain they possess (sulfhydryl chain in captopril, phosphinyl chain for fosinopril, and carboxyl for all the others), and by their lipid solubility. The last characteristic also affects their penetration into tissue.

15.2.2 **Mechanism of action**

By blocking the effect of ACE on angiotensin I, the ACEI inhibit the formation of angiotensin II. Angiotensin II is a potent vasoconstrictor and also causes salt and water retention both by actions via aldosterone and by activation of the sympathetic nervous system. Box 15.1 lists some of the other effects of angiotensin II on the body. Thus, blocking the formation of angiotensin II helps to control blood pressure. However, it is observed that this fall in plasma angiotensin II levels lasts only for several weeks. This could be due to regeneration of angiotensin II by non-ACE pathways. Under normal circumstances, angiotensin II inhibits the formation of renin. When its levels fall low, there could be a point where it is too low to inhibit renin and thereby, renin and consequently angiotensin I levels may rise. Alternate pathway enzymes such as chymases, etc. could then cleave the angiotensin I to form angiotensin II.

By six months, the levels of angiotensin II have usually returned to normal, although the blood pressure remains controlled. This is in part due to the increased levels of bradykinin (which normally would have been broken down by ACE) which is a potent vasodilator. Bradykinins also stimulate the production of nitric oxide which is a potent vasodilator. Non-steroidal anti-inflammatory drugs can blunt the blood-pressure-lowering effect of ACEI principally by blocking prostaglandin pathways in the kidneys.

ACEIs also reduce activity of the sympathetic nervous system. Although they do not consistently reduce resting plasma catecholamine concentrations, they tend to blunt reflex sympathetic activation seen with other vasodilating drugs. By causing peripheral vasodilatation, these drugs also reduce cardiac preload and afterload by their systemic vasodilatation. Their effect on heart rate is minimal even though they appear to have some inhibitory effect on the sympathetic nervous system.

Box 15.1 Effects of angiotensin II

Heart
- Myocardial hypertrophy
- Interstitial fibrosis

Coronary arteries
- Endothelial dysfunction
- Vasoconstriction of the coronaries
- Promotion of inflammation and atheroma formation

Kidneys
- Increased intraglomerular pressure
- Increased protein leak
- Glomerular growth and fibrosis
- Increased sodium reabsorption

Adrenals
- Increased formation of aldosterone

Blood
- Hypercoagulable state

ACEI also prevents the cardiac remodelling that is seen with long-term hypertension and heart failure and appears to cause regression of left ventricular hypertrophy (LVH) that is seen in hypertension. It is thought that this is primarily due to the inhibition of angiotensin II and aldosterone, both of which stimulate smooth muscle and fibrous hyperplasia.

ACEIs also have been shown to improve endothelial function and platelet function in hypertensive patients, an effect that is thought to be over and above that affected by blood pressure reductions alone.

15.3 Clinical uses

15.3.1 Use in hypertension

The efficacy of ACEI in lowering blood pressure has been well established since the early 1980s in clinical trials against placebo and has been shown to be at least as effective as other agents. However, there are conflicting data on whether it is better than other antihypertensive agents in preventing cardiovascular events and target organ damage. Early studies such as the second Swedish Trial in Old Patients with hypertension (STOP-2), the Appropriate Blood Pressure Control in Diabetes trial (ABCD), and the Captopril Prevention Project (CAPP) did not demonstrate a benefit of ACEI over other agents in preventing cardiovascular outcomes.

In a meta-analysis by the Blood Pressure Lowering Treatment Trialists Collaboration, the overview of placebo-controlled trials of ACEI (four trials, 12 124 patients, mostly with coronary heart disease) revealed reductions in stroke (30%), coronary heart disease (20%), and major cardiovascular events (21%). In the trials comparing ACEI-based regimens with diuretic-based or beta-blocker-based regimens, there were no detectable differences between randomized groups in the risks of any of the outcomes studied. For heart failure, there was a trend of borderline significance towards reduced risk among those assigned to ACEI-based therapy.

The second Australian National Blood Pressure Study (ANBP-2) compared the outcomes of 6083 hypertensive patients receiving either enalapril or hydrochlorothiazide. Addition of other agents was recommended in both to achieve good blood pressure control. In spite of identical blood pressure reduction after a follow-up period of 4.1 years, the cumulative rate of death and cardiovascular events were significantly lower in the enalapril group, which was mainly due to a decrease in myocardial infarctions. In the Anglo Scandinavian Cardiac Outcomes Trial (ASCOT), a regimen of amlodipine with perindopril was compared with atenolol and a thiazide diuretic. The study involved nearly 20 000 patients. There was no significant difference in the end point of non-fatal myocardial infarction or fatal coronary heart disease, but there was a significant difference in the secondary endpoints of all-cause mortality and fatal and non-fatal strokes.

Different results were observed in the Antihypertensive and Lipid-Lowering Treatment to Prevent Heart Attack Trial (ALLHAT), a randomized clinical trial in 33 357 hypertensives with at least one other cardiovascular risk factor. Patients were divided into three groups to receive chlortalidone, amlodipine, or lisinopril. After a mean follow-up of 4.9 years, there was no difference in the primary outcomes of cardiovascular death or non-fatal myocardial infarction. However, lisinopril had higher six-year rates of combined cardiovascular disease (33.3% vs 30.9%); stroke (6.3% vs 5.6%); and heart failure (8.7% vs 7.7%). The study, however, has been criticized for many problems with the methodology and its early termination.

Studies have also demonstrated that people of black descent may not respond well to ACEI because of low circulating renin levels in this population. However, further studies have shown that when a diuretic is added, or if the dose is increa-sed, there is substantial blood pressure-lowering effect even in this population.

15.3.2 Secondary prevention and high risk of cardiovascular disease

In the Perindopril Protection against Recurrent Stroke Study (PROGRESS) 6105 hypertensive and non-hypertensive patients with a history of stroke or transient ischaemic attack were randomly assigned perindopril or placebo. After a follow-up of four years, perindopril reduced the incidence of stroke (10% vs 14%) and also the risk of total major vascular events. The reduction of stroke was similar in hypertensives and normotensives. Combination therapy with perindopril and indapamide produced larger blood pressure reductions and larger risk reductions (43%) than did single-drug therapy with perindopril alone.

Whether ACEIs also provide benefit to patients with coronary artery disease in the absence of congestive heart failure via an anti-atherosclerotic mechanism has been investigated in several studies. Studies such as the Quinapril Ischemic Event Trial (QUIET) and the Simvastatin/Enalapril Coronary Atherosclerosis (SCAT) Trial were negative in that ACEIs failed to reduce the severity of coronary lesions on angiography as compared with placebo. However, studies such as the Heart Outcomes Prevention Evaluation Study (HOPE), the European trial On Reduction of Cardiac Events with Perindopril in Stable Coronary Artery Disease (EUROPA), the Prevention of Events with Angiotensin-Converting Enzyme Inhibition (PEACE), and the Telmisartan Alone and in Combination with Ramipril Global Endpoint Trial (ONTARGET) trials demonstrated a benefit in reducing overall cardiovascular endpoints with the use of ACEI for secondary prevention. Taken in conjunction with the trials in heart failure and after myocardial infarction, these studies argue persuasively for a general vascular protective effect of ACEI in patients with coronary and other forms of atherosclerotic arterial disease.

15.3.3 Diabetic nephropathy

In diabetic individuals, the blood pressure aims are lower than in non-diabetic patients. Both diabetes and hypertension are associated with insulin resistance. Both high-dose thiazides and beta blockers can impair insulin sensitivity in non-diabetic hypertensive individuals. In type 1 diabetic nephropathy, ACEIs have been shown to reduce proteinuria and protect against progressive glomerular sclerosis and loss of renal function. However, in type 2 diabetic nephropathy, most of the studies involve the use of angiotensin receptor blockers, although one could hypothesize that ACEI also would be effective in this setting.

15.3.4 Heart failure

The benefits of ACEI in heart failure are well established. Various trials such as the CONSENSUS with enalapril, SAVE with captopril, TRACE with trandolapril, and AIRE with ramipril have demonstrated its efficacy in treating left ventricular dysfunction both in the acute post-myocardial infarct setting and even in the non-infarct related heart failure setting. ACEIs have also been shown to cause regression of LVH in patients with hypertension, thus reducing the amount of diastolic dysfunction that might be present in these patients.

15.3.5 Atrial fibrillation

Some studies have shown a significant reduction in the incidence of atrial fibrillation with ACE inhibitors. In patients with left ventricular dysfunction caused by acute myocardial infarction, trandolapril, compared with placebo, was associated with a 47% relative risk reduction in the incidence of atrial fibrillation. In a retrospective analysis of patients with left ventricular dysfunction enrolled in the Studies Of Left Ventricular Dysfunction (SOLVD) study, enalapril, relative to placebo, was associated with a 78% risk reduction in the incidence of atrial fibrillation. In that study, enalapril was the most powerful predictor of decreased risk of atrial fibrillation. A similar finding was noted in a substudy of the Trandolapril Cardiac Evaluation (TRACE) study, where trandolapril was found to reduce the incidence of atrial fibrillation in patients with impaired left ventricular function following an acute myocardial infarction.

A study by Zaman and colleagues (2005) looked into the effects of ACE inhibitors on patients undergoing DC cardioversion for atrial fibrillation. They showed that the number of defibrillation attempts required to restore sinus rhythm and the incidence rate ratio of readmissions for atrial fibrillation were significantly lower in patients treated with ACE inhibitors. They also showed that signal-averaged P-wave duration, which is prolonged in atrial fibrillation, significantly shortens with ACE inhibitors.

Even though the exact mechanism by which ACE inhibitors reduce the risk of AF development in patients with LV dysfunction is unknown, most patients with AF have other risk factors for cardiovascular disease (CVD), including hypertension. ACE inhibitors would be a wise choice for treatment in such patients.

15.4 Side effects

In general, ACEIs are among the best-tolerated agents used to treat hypertension. In the early 1980s with high doses of ACE inhibition, many severe dose-related side effects were observed such as neutropenia, renal disease with proteinuria, skin rash, etc., but dose reduction reduced these side effects to a large extent. Non-specific complaints such as lethargy, headache, fatigue, nausea, and diarrhoea have been reported. The most common side effects include the following:

- First-dose hypotension
- Dry, hacking, non-productive cough
- Blunting of normal compensatory responses to volume depletion
- Mild worsening of renal functions (up to 20% of increase of the baseline renal parameters is expected and acceptable)
- Hyperkalaemia

Rare side effects include angioedema, anaphylactoid reactions, leukopenia, and taste distur-bances along with severe renal insufficiency. Significant worsening of renal functions should alert one to the possibility of renal artery stenosis.

15.5 Contraindications

Absolute contraindications include pregnancy, bilateral renal artery stenosis, or unilateral ste-nosis in a solitary kidney. A history of previous angioneurotic oedema especially associated with prior ACEI use is also an absolute contraindication. Relative contraindications include severe renal insufficiency and aortic stenosis and obstructive cardiomyopathy.

15.6 Current recommendations

As per the British Hypertension Society guidelines and the European society of Cardiology (2013), the compelling indications for ACEI include heart failure, LV dysfunction post-myocardial infarction or established coronary heart disease, presence of type 1 diabetic nephropathy, and secondary prevention of strokes. Possible indications include chronic renal failure, type 2 dia-betic nephropathy, and proteinuric renal disease. The recommendations also suggest that these drugs be used as first-line monotherapy in patients who are below the age of 55 and those not of African-Caribbean descent. They are best avoided in a combination with other blockers of the renin angiotensin system such as angiotensin receptor blockers or renin inhibitors. Studies such as the ACCOMPLISH trial have demonstrated that they work well in combination with calcium-channel blockers. They are also recommended in patients with LVH.

Key references

Bakris GL, Serafidis PA, Weir MR, *et al.* for the ACCOMPLISH Trial Investigators (2010). Renal outcomes with different fixed-dose combination therapies in patients with hypertension at high risk for cardiovas-cular events (ACCOMPLISH): a prespecified secondary analysis of randomised controlled trial. *Lancet*; 375: 1173–81.

Blood Pressure Lowering Treatment Trialists' Collaboration (2000). Effects of ACE inhibitors, calcium antagonists and other blood pressure lowering drugs: results of prospectively designed overviews of randomised trials. *Lancet*; 355: 1955–64.

Blood Pressure Lowering Treatment Trialists' Collaboration (2003). Effects of different blood-pressure-lowering regimens on major cardiovascular events: results of prospectively-designed overviews of randomised trials. *Lancet*; 362: 1527–35.

Blood Pressure Lowering Treatment Trialists' Collaboration (2005). Effects of different blood-pressure-lowering regimens on major cardiovascular events in individuals with and without diabetes mellitus: results of prospectively-designed overviews of randomised trials. *Archives of Internal Medicine*; 165: 1410–19.

Fox KM; EURopean trial On reduction of cardiac events with Perindopril in stable coronary Artery dis-ease Investigators (2003). Efficacy of perindopril in reduction of cardiovascular events among patients with stable coronary artery disease: randomised, double-blind, placebo-controlled, multicentre trial (the EUROPA study). *Lancet*; 362(9386): 782–88.

Kunz R, Friedrich C, Wolbers M, *et al.* (2008) Meta-analysis: effect of monotherapy and combination therapy with inhibitors of the renin angiotensin system on proteinuria in renal disease. *Annals of Internal Medicine*; 148: 30–48.

Reboldi G, Angeli F, Cavallini C, *et al.* (2008). Comparison between angiotensin-converting enzyme inhibitors and angiotensin receptor blockers on the risk of myocardial infarction, stroke and death: a meta-analysis. *Journal of Hypertension*; 26: 1282–89.

Regulski M, Regulska K, Stainsz BJ, *et al.* (2014). Chemistry and Pharmacology of Angiotensin converting enzyme inhibitors. *Current Pharmacological Design*; November 12 (epub)

Schneider MP, Hua TA, Bohm M, *et al.* (2010). Prevention of atrial fibrillation by renin-angiotensin system inhibition: a meta-analysis. *Journal of the American College of Cardiology*; 55: 2299–307.

Shahin Y, Khan JA, Chetter I (2012). Angiotensin converting enzyme inhibitors effect on arterial stiffness and wave reflections: a meta-analysis and meta-regression of randomised controlled trials. *Atherosclerosis*; 221: 18–33.

The Heart Outcomes Prevention Evaluation (HOPE) investigators (2000). Effects of an angiotensin-converting-enzyme inhibitor, ramipril, on cardiovascular events in high-risk patients. *New England Journal of Medicine*; 342: 145–53.

The Task Force for the management of arterial hypertension of the European Society of Hypertension (ESH) and of the European Society of Cardiology (2013). ESH/ESC Guidelines for the management of arterial hypertension. *European Heart Journal*; 34, 2159–219.

Chapter 16

Angiotensin receptor blockers and hypertension

Mehmood Butt

> ## Key points
>
> - The pharmacological management of hypertension involves modulating the renin–angiotensin–aldosterone system at various molecular sites.
> - There are two main receptors for angiotensin II—angiotensin 1 (AT1) and angiotensin 2 (AT2) receptors.
> - Angiotensin receptor blockers mainly inhibit AT1 receptors.
> - Angiotensin receptor blockers have an established role in both primary and secondary disease prevention—in particular, in patients with hypertension and heart failure.

16.1 Background

16.1.1 Pharmacology

With the identification and understanding of the renin–angiotensin–aldosterone system (RAAS) and its pivotal role in hypertension, there has been considerable research into modulating its pathways at different molecular sites. Of particular importance is the development of angiotensin receptor blockers (ARBs) to inhibit the final pathway within this negative feedback loop.

Saralasin (sar 1 Ile8-ANG II) was the first ARB introduced into clinical practice in early 1970s. Due to its peptide-based structure, it was unsuitable for oral administration and had poor pharmacokinetic properties (i.e. poor bioavailability, short duration of action). Second-generation non-peptide ARBs had imidazole rings and had more desirable characteristics such as oral administration and greater sensitivity for angiotensin II receptors. Thereafter, second-generation ARBs were further modified by substituting the imidazole rings with heterocyclic rings, creating agents with even greater affinity for the AT1 receptor. This has led to the manufacture of the new-generation ARBs, all collectively named with the suffix 'sartan'.

16.1.2 Angiotensin II receptors

Two main classes of angiotensin II receptors—angiotensin 1 (AT1) and angiotensin 2 (AT2)—have been identified in both animal and human models.

In the rodent model, AT1 receptors have been sub-classified into AT1a and AT1b receptors. AT1a receptors are abundant in vascular smooth muscles whilst the AT1b receptors are predominantly present in the pituitary gland, adrenals, and periventricular cerebral areas. It is therefore postulated that the AT1a receptors play a major role in the regulation of vascular tone, and the AT1b receptors are responsible for hormonal control and osmotic regulation. In contrast to AT1, AT2 receptors remain poorly understood appear to be present mainly in foetal tissue, distinct brain areas, the adrenals, ovaries, and uterus. It is postulated that AT2 receptors play a role in cell regulation.

16.2 **Mechanisms of action: RAAS revisited**

With the multifactorial stimulation of the RAAS within the kidney (reduced renal sodium, reduced renal perfusion pressure, and B-1 receptor stimulation), renin is released form the juxtaglomerular apparatus. Renin acts to convert circulating angiotensinogen (produced by the lungs) to angiotensin I. Further conversion of angiotensin I to angiotensin II is mediated through angiotensin-converting enzyme (ACE), and in turn angiotensin II stimulates the blood pressure regulatory mechanisms through the activation of AT1 and AT2 receptors and aldosterone secretion form the adrenal cortex.

In particular, it is the angiotensin 1 (AT1) receptor that has the most profound effect on increasing blood pressure through stimulating vasoconstriction, renal sodium resorption, and further sympathetic nervous system activation. By the direct antagonism of the angiotensin receptors, ARBs avoid the inhibition of ACE, which in turn prevents the build up of bradykinins, which are responsible for the dry cough experienced by some patients taking ACE inhibitors. Therefore, ARBs provide a specific inhibitory effect on the RAAS system whilst avoiding some of the side effects experienced with ACE inhibitors.

A schematic representation of the RAAS system is shown in Figure 16.1.

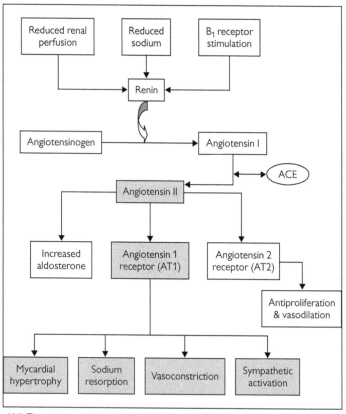

Figure 16.1 The renin–angiotensin–aldosterone system (RAAS)

Table 16.1 Pharmacological properties of angiotensin receptor blockers

Drug	Bioavailability	Food effect	Active metabolite	Plasma half-life (h)	Protein binding (%)	AT1 receptor affinity	Mode of antagonism
Losartan	33	Minimal	Y	2	98.7	50	C
Valsartan	25	40–50% reduction	N	6	95.0	10	NC
candesartan cilexetil	42	N	Y	3.5–4	99.5	280	–
Irbesartan	70	N	N	11–15	>90	5	NC
Eprosartan	13	N	N	5–9	97.0	100	C
Telmisartan	40–60	N	N	24	>99.5	10	NC
Olmesartan	26	N	Y	12–18	99.0	–	NC

Adapted from Aulakh et al., *Life sciences*. 2007.

Y = Yes, N = No, C = Competitive, NC = Non-competitive.

Affinity parameters (Affinity of 1 = greatest affinity for AT1 receptor).

Table 16.2 Indications for ARBs		
Class of drug	Compelling indication	Possible indications
ARBs	• ACE inhibitor intolerance • Type 2 diabetic nephropathy • Hypertension with LVH • Heart failure in ACE inhibitor intolerant patients • Post MI	• LV dysfunction post MI • Other antihypertensive therapy intolerance • Proteinuric renal disease • Chronic renal disease • Heart failure

From BHS IV Guidelines, *Journal of Human Hypertension*. 2004.
ACE = angiotensin converting enzyme, LVH = left ventricular hypertrophy, MI = myocardial infarction

16.3 **The pharmacological differences between angiotensin receptor blockers**

A number of ARBs have now been developed and although they all exhibit a high selectivity for the angiotensin II receptors, they vary in their properties such as the affinity for the AT1/AT2 receptors, bioavailability, mode of antagonism, and the second messenger signalling induced at the cellular level. Table 16.1 summarizes some of the pharmacological differences between the ARBs.

16.4 **The British Hypertension Society (BHS) guidelines**

ARBs are well established in the BHS guidelines on hypertension management. They are part of the 'A' treatment algorithm and may be used as a first-line therapy although this is usually in the context of ACE inhibitor intolerance. The ARBs have been extensively investigated both in primary and secondary disease prevention with promising results. Therefore, the BHS has also issued guidance on the indications for ARB use, which is summarized in Table 16.2.

16.5 **Clinical role of angiotensin receptor blockers**

16.5.1 **Patients with hypertension**

The role of ARBs in patients with hypertension alone has been investigated in three principal randomized controlled trials—the Losartan Intervention For Endpoint Reduction in Hypertension (LIFE), The Study of COgnition and Prognosis in the Elderly (SCOPE), and the Valsartan Antihypertensive Long-term Use Evaluation (VALUE) trials—summarized in Table 16.3.

The LIFE trial compared losartan with atenolol in 9193 patients. The losartan-treated group had a 13% lower adjusted risk of the primary composite end point (cardiovascular mortality, myocardial infarction (MI), and stroke) compared to atenolol, although the observed blood pressure reductions were similar in both study arms.

The SCOPE trial compared candesartan to placebo with standard therapy in 4964 patients. Although there was no difference between the treatment groups for the primary endpoint, patients treated with candesartan were observed to have a 27.8% and 23.6% reduction in both non-fatal stroke and all-cause stroke, respectively.

The VALUE trial investigated the efficacy of valsartan compared to amlodipine in 15 245 patients with hypertension and a high risk of cardiovascular disease. In contrast to LIFE and

Table 16.3 Clinical trials of angiotensin receptor blockers in patients with hypertension

Study	Therapy	Results
LIFE	Losartan 50–100 mg/day v atenolol 50–100 mg/day Follow-up duration: 4.8 years	1) Same BP reductions in both groups 2) Losartan reduced adjusted risk of composite primary endpoint (CV mortality, MI, and stroke) by 13% ($p = 0.021$) 3) Lower incidence of new-onset diabetes in losartan group
SCOPE	Candesartan 8–16 mg/day vs. placebo + standard therapy Follow-up duration: 3.7 years	1) Greater BP reduction observed in candesartan group. 2) Candesartan group had reduced non-fatal stoke (27.8%, $p = 0.04$) and all cause stroke (23.6%, $p = 0.056$).
VALUE	Valsartan 80–160 mg/day vs amlodipine 5–10 mg/day Follow-up duration: 4.2 years	1) BP reduction observed in both groups, but greater reduction in the amlodipine group. 2) No difference observed for the composite outcome (sudden cardiac death, MI, heart failure admission, death from coronary intervention).

LVH = left ventricular hypertrophy, MI = myocardial infarction, BP = blood pressure.

SCOPE, there was a greater reduction in blood pressure in the amlodipine group, the effects being more pronounced in the earlier stages of the trial. Furthermore, the primary composite end point (sudden cardiac death, MI, hospitalization for heart failure, or death due to coronary intervention) was similar between the two groups.

16.5.2 **Patients with renal disease**

Microalbuminuria is a marker of cardiovascular disease and early renal dysfunction. Therefore, pharmacological agents that can delay the progression of microalbuminuria and renal disease may have cardiovascular benefits, at least by lessening the systemic effects of renal pathology. There have been several randomized controlled trials investigating the efficacy of ARBs in patients with renal disease including the following:

- The CHILI T2D study
- The Diabetics Exposed to Telmisartan And enalapriL study group (DETAIL) trial
- The Irbesartan Diabetic Nephropathy Trial (IDNT)
- The IRbesartan in Patients with Type 2 Diabetes and MicroalbuminuriA 2 (IRMA-2) trial
- The Microalbuminuria Reduction with VALsartan (MARVAL) trial
- The Reduction of Endpoints in NIDDM with the Angiotensin II Antagonist Losartan (RENAAL) trial

These trials included over 4000 patients with diabetes and diabetic nephropathy, and have shown numerous benefits including a risk reduction of developing progressive diabetic nephropathy and end-stage renal disease. The benefits favour the use of ARBs in comparison to both placebo and alternative antihypertensive agents.

The much more recent Ongoing Telmisartan Alone and In combination with Ramipril Global Endpont Trial (ONTARGET) study and the Telmisartan Randomized Assessment Study in Angiotensin-Converting-Enzyme-Inhibitor Intolerant Subjects with Cardiovascular Disease

(TRANSCEND) trials studied the impact of Telmisartan either on its own or in combination with an ACE inhibitor. It showed that they might have additional benefits on cardiovascular protection in combination, especially in high risk patients, but they do so at a higher risk of renal impairment.

16.5.3 Patients with heart failure

There have been many randomized trials evaluating the efficacy of ARBs in patients with heart failure including the following:

- NAGOYA-HEART study—valsartan versus amlodipine (favours valsartan in mortality reduction)
- The Candesartan in Heart Reduction in Mortality and Morbidity (CHARM) trial—candesartan versus placebo (favours ARB)
- The Losartan Heart Failure Survival Study (ELITE II)—losartan versus captopril (no significant difference found)
- The Valsartan Heart Failure Trial (Val-HeFT)
- The VALsartan In Acute Myocardial INfarction Trial (VALIANT)
- The OPtimal Trial in Myocardial Infarction with the Angiotensin II Antagonist Losartan (OPTIMAAL)

ARBs have been compared with ACE inhibitors as well. The VALIANT trial concluded non-inferiority of valsartan compared to captopril. Similarly, the OPTIMAAL trial did not show significant difference between losartan and captopril, although the ARB was better tolerated.

These studies have clearly established the clinical efficacy of ARBs to reduce both morbidity and mortality in patients with heart failure. Improvements in NYHA class, ejection fraction, and quality of life were observed with the sub-studies of some of the trials.

16.6 Safety of ARBs

The ARBs have a better safety profile compared with the ACE inhibitors (avoidance of an ACE inhibitor induced cough and less incidence of angioedema). However, just like ACE inhibitors, ARBs may have detrimental effect on renal profile and hence close bioochemical monitoring is recommended (especially in diabetics, patients with peripheral vascular disease, and patient who have existing renal impairment). Combined use with ACE inhibitor has not shown any clinical benefits in clinical trials. ARBs are contraindicated for use in pregnancy.

Key references

Aulakh GK, Sodhi RK, Singh M (2007). An update on non-peptide angiotensin receptor antagonists and related RAAS modulators. *Life Sciences*; 81: 615–39.

Basile JN, Chrysant S (2006). The importance of early antihypertensive efficacy: the role of angiotensin II receptor blocker therapy. *Journal of Human Hypertension*; 20(3): 169–75.

Chung O, Unger T (1993). Pharmacology of angiotensin receptors and AT1 receptor blockers. *Basic Research in Cardiology*; 93(Suppl 2): 15–23.

Kendall MJ (1998). Therapeutic advantages of AT1 blockers in hypertension. *Basic Research in Cardiology*, 93(Suppl 2): 47–50.

Nickenig G, Ostergren J, Struijker-Boudier H (2006). Clinical evidence for the cardiovascular benefits of angiotensin receptor blockers. *Journal of the Renin–Angiotensin–Aldosterone System*; 7(Suppl 1): S1–7.

Sleight P, Redon J, Verdacchia P, *et al.* (2009). Prognostic value of Blood pressure in patients with high vascular risk in the Ongoing Telmisartan Alone and In combination with Ramipril Global Endpoint trial study (ONTRAGET). *Journal of Hypertension*; 27(7):1360–9.

Tobe SW, Clase CM, Gao P (2011). Cardiovascular and renal outcomes with telmisartan, ramipril, or both in people at high renal risk: results from the ONTARGET and TRANSCEND studies..*Circulation*; 123(10):1098–107.

Turnbull F, Blood Pressure Lowering Treatment Trialists' Collaboration. (2003). Effects of different blood-pressure-lowering regimens on major cardiovascular events: results of prospectively-designed overviews of randomised trials. *Lancet;* 362: 1527–35.

Chapter 17

Other antihypertensives

Shankar BG Patil and Muzahir H Tayebjee

Key points

- Since 2007, only two new antihypertensives have been licensed—aliskerin and azilsartan medoxomil.
- Other conventional antihypertensive drugs currently used are alpha-adrenoreceptor antagonists, centrally acting agents, vasodilators, and aldosterone receptor antagonists.
- Further understanding of the role of renin–angiotensin–aldosterone system (RAAS), endothelins, vasopeptidases, and natriuretic peptide agonists in the pathophysiology of blood pressure regulation has been key to the development of novel agents.

119

17.1 Introduction

Alpha-adrenoreceptor antagonists, centrally acting agents, vasodilators, and aldosterone receptor antagonist have roles in resistant hypertension and in specific sub-groups of hypertensive patients. This chapter covers the pharmacology and indications for these agents.

17.2 Alpha-adrenoreceptor antagonists (alpha blockers)

Alpha-adrenoreceptors (α_1 and α_2) are widely distributed on vascular smooth muscle cells. α_1 receptors predominantly mediate vasoconstriction and blocking these results in non-specific arterial and venous dilatation and consequent blood pressure (BP) reduction.

The main indications include:

- Selective alpha blockers (prazosin, doxazosin, terazosin) can be used as add-on therapy for uncontrolled hypertension (ASCOT trial) and benign prostatic hypertrophy.
- Non selective alpha blockers (phenoxybenzamine, phentolamine) are used to treat hypertension associated with proven phaeochromocytoma.

The main side effects are dizziness, orthostatic hypotension, nasal congestion, somnolence, headache, and reflex tachycardia. They tend to cause fluid retention and should be avoided in heart failure.

When used as first line of treatment for hypertension, patients had a higher risk of cardiovascular events in two major clinical trials, ALLHAT and Veterans Administration Study.

17.3 Centrally acting agents

Central BP regulation is mediated via alpha adrenoreceptors located in the pons and medulla. Centrally acting agents cross the blood–brain barrier and act on post synaptic $\alpha2$ receptors, reducing brainstem sympathetic outflow and thereby causing peripheral vasodilatation and lowering blood pressure. They include methyldopa and imidazolidine-related compounds like clonidine and guanfacine.

The main indications are

- Mainly as add-on therapy in resistant hypertension
- hypertension in pregnancy (alpha methy-dopa)
- hypertensive emergencies

The main side effects are postural hypotension, bradycardia, dry mouth, sexual impotence, haemolytic anaemia (positive Coomb's test), extrapyramidal disorders, hepatitis, sedation, withdrawal phenomenon, and tolerance.

Patients on phosphodiesterase-5 inhibitors (sildenafil, tadalafil) should avoid alpha blockers as this may result in profound hypotension.

17.4 **Vasodilators (nitrates)**

Vasodilators act directly on vascular endothelium via nitric oxide release which stimulates cyclic guanosine monophosphate-(cGMP)-mediated vascular smooth muscle relaxation and vasodilatation.

The main indications are:

- Predominantly hypertensive emergencies (sodium nitroprusside, nitroglycerine)
- Refractory hypertension

The main side effects include headache, cutaneous flushing, hypotension, tachycardia, and angina. Prolonged sodium nitroprusside use can cause thiocyanate toxicity.

When used alone, they can stimulate baroreceptors leading to reflex tachycardia, rise in cardiac output, and increased cardiac contraction. This can trigger angina. Hence, they should be combined with beta-adrenergic blockers.

17.5 **Novel antihypertensive drugs**

The various newer antihypertensive agents have been summarized in Table 17.1.

These are mainly agents that act on the RAAS. The mode of action of these agents is shown in Figure 17.1.

17.5.1 **Renin inhibitors**

Renin (angiotensinase) is a proteolytic enzyme released by renal juxtaglomerular cells in response to low arterial blood pressure and low sodium (Na) delivery to the macula densa. Renin acts on plasma angiotensinogen (synthesized by the liver) to angiotensin I which ultimately leads to the production of angiotensin II and aldosterone. Renin inhibitors inhibit the conversion of angiotensinogen to angiotensin I.

The first- and second-generation peptide-like renin inhibitors were ineffective due to poor bioavailability and lack of potency. Aliskiren is the first orally bioavailable third generation non-peptide renin inhibitor approved for treatment of hypertension. It reduces plasma renin activity by 75%. Three surrogate outcome studies on aliskiren have shown it to be as effective as ACE-I, ARBs, calcium-channel blockers (CCB), and diuretics in controlling BP, heart failure, and proteinuria. Fourth-generation renin inhibitors are being developed with improved bioavailability and safety profile.

Table 17.1 Novel antihypertensive drugs

Class	Name	Dose	Main indications	Side effects
Renin inhibitors	Aliskiren	150–300 mg/d	Hypertension	Angioedema, hyperkalaemia, hypotension, diarrhoea, rash, gout, renal stones.
Aldosterone Blockers	Spironolactone	50–400 mg/d	Mineralocorticoid hypertension, congestive heart failure, essential hypertension	Gynaecomastia, hyperkalaemia, diarrhoea, menstrual irregularity.
	Eplerenone	25–200 mg/d	Essential hypertension, hypertension associated with left ventricular hypertrophy, congestive heart failure following myocardial infarction	Headache, dizziness, angina, abnormal vaginal bleeding, hypercholesterolaemia, hypertriglyceridaemia, diarrhoea, abdominal pain.
AT1R receptor receptor antagonist	Azilsartan medoxomil	40–80 mg/d	Essential hypertension alone or in combination with others	Cough, nausea, fatigue, muscle spasm, postural dizziness.
*Aldosterone synthase inhibitors	LC1699		Phase-II trials are ongoing in patients of hypertension with	
Vasopeptidase inhibitor	Omapatrilat	10–40 mg/d	Hypertension, congestive heart failure (in trials)	Angioedema.
Soluble epoxide hydrolase inhibitors	AR9821			

* Awaiting phase1 and 2 studies.

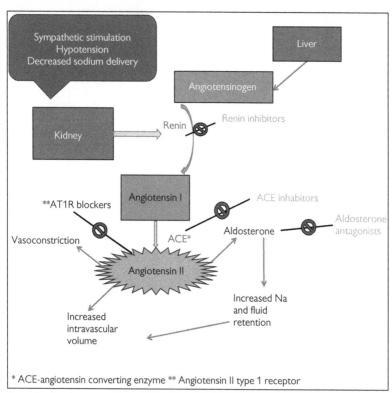

Figure 17.1 RAAS (renin–angiotensin–aldosterone system)

They are currently approved for monotherapy and combination therapy.

They are not recommended as first-line treatment and currently not in the NICE guidelines.

The main side effects are diarrhoea, hyperkalaemia, angioedema, and raised creatinine kinase.

The co-administration of aliskiren with ACE inhibiors and ARBs was associated with increased incidence of renal impairment, hyperkalaemia, and hypotension in diabetic patients. The FDA and MHRA have issued a warning to combination therapy in patients with moderate to severe renal failure (eGFR < 60 ml/min).

17.5.2 **Aldosterone-receptor blockers**

Aldosterone is synthesized by the kidneys in response to angiotensin II and acts on mineralo-corticoid receptors situated in the heart, vasculature and kidneys. It increases blood pressure by acting on the distal renal tubules, increasing water and sodium re-absorption. Aldosterone also has profibrotic effects resulting in tissue inflammation, cardiac fibrosis, and glomeruloscle-rosis. Aldosterone-receptor blockers therefore attenuate these processes.

Spironolactone and eplerenone are two currently used aldosterone-receptor blocker drugs.

Spironolactone is a steroidal anti-mineralocorticoid with non-specific oestrogen and gluco-corticoid effects and is approved for treating resistant hypertension

Eplerenone is a selective mineralocorticoid blocker and lacks antiandrogenic or progestational side effects. Eplerenone is currently licensed in UK for treating post myocardial infarction heart failure. In US and Japan, it is licensed for treating hypertension.

The main side effects are renal failure, hyperkalemia, and gynaecomastia.

17.5.3 Angiotensin II type 1 receptor (AT1R) blockers

AT1R receptor is an angiotensin II type 1 receptor that regulates aldosterone synthesis and acts predominantly as a vasopressor. Azilsartan is the only AT1R blocker approved for hypertension. In a trial of nearly 6000 patients, azilsartan 40–80 mg/d was compared with placebo and active comparator (valsartan 320 mg/d or olmesartan 40 mg/d) and was shown to be superior to olmesartan 40 mg (−5 mmHg) and valsartan 320 mg (−3 mmHg) in lowering the mean 24-hour ambulatory and clinic blood pressure that was sustained over a period of 26 weeks.

It is currently approved for treatment of hypertension in US as both monotherapy and in combination with chlortalidone, a thiazide-like diuretic.

Despite their efficacy, data on long-term outcomes are not yet available.

17.5.4 Aldosterone synthase inhibitors

Targeting aldosterone synthesis to prevent the deleterious effects of angiotensin II has resulted in research on novel agents for resistant hypertension. The reactive increase in aldosterone levels as a result of inhibiting the aldosterone receptor could be counteracted by aldosterone synthase inhibitors, LCI 699 is the first aldosterone synthase inhibitor, with phase II studies showing good pressure-lowering effect (−7.1 mmHg) with a dose of 1 mg twice daily compared with placebo. It does not prevent epithelial adverse effects such as sodium retention and potassium excretion mediated by aldosterone. Hence, there is a search for aldosterone synthase inhibitors with greater specificity.

17.5.5 Natriuretic peptide receptor agonists (NPRA)

Atrial natriuretic peptide (ANP) and brain natriuretic peptide (BNP) refer to peptides that induce natriuresis and vasodilatation. ANP is produced in response to atrial myocyte stretch and acts on the ANP receptors in renal, vascular, and cardiac tissues. Their major role is to counteract the vasopressor effects of aldosterone.

PL3994, an NPRA has shown blood pressure-lowering effect and natriuresis in healthy volunteers in phase 1 trials. In phase IIa clinical trials, combining PL3994 with ACE inhibitors produced a pronounced blood pressure reduction suggesting a synergistic effect. Further clinical trials are awaited for full clinical effects and adverse events.

17.5.6 Soluble epoxide hydrolase inhibitors (sEH inhibitors)

sEH is an enzyme expressed in various tissues including liver and vascular endothelium. It hydrolyses endogenous lipid epoxides, preventing them from exerting their vasodilatory effects. Inhibiting sEH causes vasodilation and lowers blood pressure.

AR9821 is the first sEH inhibitor that is being investigated in clinical trials. In animal models it lowered blood pressure, improved vascular function, and reduced renal damage in rats with angiotensin II-induced hypertension. However, a phase I clinical trial in healthy volunteers failed to show any blood pressure-lowering effect. In a separate study, it lowered the activity of sHE in patients with hypertension and diabetes indicating a possible role in specific group of patients.

17.5.7 Vasopeptidase inhibitors (VPI)

VPIs inhibit both ACE and neutral endopeptidases (NEP). NEP is an endothelial cell-surface zinc metallopeptidase involved in degradation of natriuretic peptides. Inhibition of NEP increases levels of natriuretic peptides and thus potentiates the blood pressure lowering effect of ACE inhibitors. They reduce vasoconstriction, improve sodium/water balance, thus decrease blood pressure and peripheral vascular resistance.

Omapatrilat, a VPI reduced systolic BP 3.6 mmHg more than enalapril in a large multicentre randomized controlled clinical trial in untreated or uncontrolled hypertension-OCTAVE. However, angioedema was more common than enalapril. Larger trials are ongoing and they may help to define further benefits and side effects.

17.6 Dual inhibitors/combinations

One-third of hypertensive patients require more than two pharmacological agents to achieve adequate blood pressure control. Current European guidelines recommend at least two antihypertensive medications for stage-II hypertension. Trials involving more than one antihypertensive drugs and heart failure trials that included additional antihypertensive medication in their treatment regimen showed reduction in mortality.

Combination therapy provides complementary benefits because each agent blocks the counterregulatory effects of the other.

Some of the combinations currently approved for clinical use/trial are AT1R blockers with vasopeptidase inhibitors, vasopeptidase inhibitors with endothelin converting enzyme inhibitors, AT1R blockers with diuretics, and aliskerin with amlodipine and hydrochlorothiazide.

References

Anandan SK, Webb HK, Chen D, et al. (2011). 1-(1-acetyl-piperidin-4-yl)-3-adamantan-1-yl-urea (AR9281) as a potent, selective, and orally available soluble epoxide hydrolase inhibitor with efficacy in rodent models of hypertension and dysglycemia. Bioorganic and Medicinal Chemistry Letters; 21(3): 983–88.

Calhoun DA, White WB, Krum H, et al. (2011). Effects of a novel aldosterone synthase inhibitor for treatment of primary hypertension: results of a randomized, double-blind, placebo- and active-controlled phase 2 trial. Circulation; 124(18): 1945–55.

Campbell DJ (2003). Vasopeptidase inhibition: a double-edged sword?" Hypertension; 41(3): 383–89.

Chapman NCL, Chang B, Dahlof PS, et al. (2008). Effect of doxazosin gastrointestinal therapeutic system as third-line antihypertensive therapy on blood pressure and lipids in the Anglo-Scandinavian Cardiac Outcomes Trial. Circulation; 118 (1):42–8.

Chen Y, Meng L, H Shao H, et al. (2013). Aliskiren vs. other antihypertensive drugs in the treatment of hypertension: a meta-analysis. Hypertension Research; 36(3): 252–61

Chrysant SG (2011). Single-pill triple-combination therapy: an alternative to multiple-drug treatment of hypertension. Postgraduate Medicine; 123(6): 21–31.

Conlin PR, Spence JD, Williams B, et al. (2000). Angiotensin II antagonists for hypertension: are there differences in efficacy? American Journal of Hypertension; 13(4 Pt 1): 418–26.

Imig JD (2009). Adenosine2A receptors and epoxyeicosatrienoic acids: a recipe for salt and blood pressure regulation. Hypertension; 54(6): 1223–25.

Jordan R, Stark J, Huskey S, et al. (2008). Phase 1 study of the novel A-type natriuretic receptor agonist, PL-3994, in healthy volunteers. Journal of Cardiac Failure; 14(6) suppl: S70.

Kostis JB, Packer M, Black HR, et al. (2004). Omapatrilat and enalapril in patients with hypertension: the Omapatrilat Cardiovascular Treatment vs. Enalapril (OCTAVE) trial. American Journal of Hypertension; 17(2): 103–11.

Marrs JC (2010). Spironolactone management of resistant hypertension. Annals of Pharmacotherapy; 44(11): 1762–69.

Wengenmayer C, Krikov M, Mueller S, et al. (2011). Novel therapy approach in primary stroke prevention: simultaneous inhibition of endothelin converting enzyme and neutral endopeptidase in spontaneously hypertensive, stroke-prone rats improves survival. Neurological Research; 33(2):201–7.

White WB, Weber MA, Sica D, et al. (2011). Effects of the angiotensin receptor blocker azilsartan medoxomil versus olmesartan and valsartan on ambulatory and clinic blood pressure in patients with stages 1 and 2 hypertension. Hypertension; 57(3): 413–20.

Chapter 18

Renal denervation

Viji Samuel Thomson

> ### Key points
>
> - Hypertension is associated with an increased sympathetic tone.
> - Manipulation of this has been tried with pharmacological methods.
> - Renal sympathetic denervation reduces the sympathetic tone in hypertensive patients and uncontrolled trials have demonstrated a decrease in blood pressure in severe resistant hypertension.
> - Caution must be applied to the widespread use of this procedure as although it is safe, a recent large randomized controlled trial has failed to show a benefit in blood pressure reduction.
> - The long-term effects of the ablation of renal sympathetic nerves is not known.

18.1 Introduction

Hypertension is a common clinical disorder with significant morbidity and mortality. The predicted number of adults with hypertension in the year 2025 is 1.56 billion. Hypertension treatment resulted in 16% reduction in mortality related to coronary heart disease, 38% reduction in stroke mortality, and 52% reduction in occurrence of congestive cardiac failure. Despite treatment with multiple drugs approximately 15–30 % of patients with hypertension do not achieve target blood pressures. Among the various factors that contribute to hypertension, an increased sympathetic tone has been known to play an important part. Drugs targeting this system (such as beta and alpha blockers) have been tried. Physical means to alter this hyper-sympathetic state have been tried experimentally in the past. Renal denervation (RDN) is a minimally invasive procedure which has shown promise to deal with difficult to treat essential hypertension patients.

18.2 Rationale of renal denervation therapy

Renal denervation for hypertension is an old concept and has been practised in the past in radical forms like bilateral nephrectomy for patients with end-stage renal disease whose blood pressures were not controlled with medications. Animal studies had already shown the efficacy of renal denervation in lowering blood pressure. Dibona and colleagues had shown that increasing renal nerve stimulation results in increased renin secretion, followed by decreased urinary sodium excretion and decrease in renal blood flow, all leading to elevation of blood pressure. Catheter ablation resulted in partial to almost complete ablation of renal sympathetic nerves, which was confirmed by a mean reduction in nor-epinephrine spill over of 47.5% compared to baseline. Thus renal sympathectomy can result in lowering of blood pressure.

18.3 **Efficacy of the procedure**

Two human studies have been undertaken, based on the above hypothesis. The first (Symplicity HTN-1 trial) is a case series consisting of 153 patients, the three-year results of which are now available. In 88 patients for whom follow-up data were available at three years, the systolic blood pressure decreased by 32 mmHg (95% CI −35.7 to −28.2). The corresponding decrease in diastolic blood pressure was 14.4 mmHg (95% CI −16.9 to −11.9), and greater than 10 mmHg drop in systolic blood pressure was observed in 93% of the patients.

In the only unblinded randomized trial available to date (Symplicity HTN-2 trial), the patients who underwent renal denervation had an impressive reduction in blood pressure of 32/12 mmHg (SD of 23/11 mmHg) at six months.

Following renal denervation, Mahmoud and colleagues demonstrated a reduction in the renal resistive index and incidence of albuminuria with no change in the glomerular filtration rate in 88 patients with resistant hypertension. The low risk of adverse events along with benefits of blood pressure lowering makes RDN a very attractive therapeutic option for patients with resistant hypertension.

18.4 **Subset of patients who may benefit from RDN**

Currently, most of the studies have targeted patients with resistant hypertension defined as patients whose blood pressure is not controlled on maximally tolerated doses of three antihypertensives of which one is a diuretic. The inclusion criteria for this therapy was based on office blood pressure recordings greater than 160/100 mmHg for non-diabetics and 150/90 mmHg for diabetics. Patients with secondary causes of hypertension were excluded. As per the joint UK Societies' consensus statement on renal denervation of resistant hypertension, patients that are beyond step 4 may be considered for this therapy after explaining the uncertainty regarding the long-term results of this procedure.

18.5 **Anatomic suitability**

In the Symplicity trial patients with accessory renal arteries, renal arteries measuring less than 4 mm, early division of renal arteries (ostium to bifurcation < 20 mm), haemodynamically significant renal artery stenosis and more than one main renal artery were excluded. The anatomic suitability was determined by MR angiography, CT angiography, or renal angiography.

18.6 **Procedure**

The procedure is percutaneously done in the catheterization laboratory by personnel proficient in interventional cardiology or radiology from the femoral approach under mild sedation. It essentially involves placing a catheter in the renal artery through the femoral artery. Six to eight low power radiofrequency applications lasting 90 seconds to two minutes are made at each location in a spiral fashion in each renal artery. The proximal portion of the renal artery 5–10 mm beyond the ostium is preferred site due to its relatively dense sympathetic innervation.

18.7 **Complications**

It is generally a safe procedure with minimal short-term complications as mentioned below. The true long-term effects are still not quite clear.

18.7.1 **Procedure related**

Immediate

1. Visceral pain relieved with analgesics (15)
2. Access site complications (6)
3. Renal artery dissection requiring stenting (6, 15)

Delayed

1. Renal artery stenosis.

    This could not be attributed due to the procedure but may be progression of natural atherosclerotic disease.

18.7.2 **Non-procedure related**

The non-procedure related complications are related to hypotension, which is remedied by reduction in the dose of antihypertensive medications. Other side effects included nausea and edema, which requires only symptomatic treatment.

18.8 **Non-responders to renal denervation**

18.8.1 **Patients with single renal arteries**

Approximately 7% of patients who undergo renal denervation do not demonstrate a reduction in blood pressure. This may suggest incomplete or insufficient sympathectomy, established target organ damage, or it may be related the duration of hypertension or age of the patient.

18.8.2 **Patients with accessory renal arteries**

Recent study by Kaltenbach and colleagues revealed a non-significant reduction in both office and mean 24-hour systolic blood pressures in a subgroup of patients who underwent denervation of all accessory renal arteries, incomplete denervation, or non-denervation of accessory renal arteries.

18.9 **Future perspectives**

RDN has been used in patients with moderate treatment resistant hypertension defined as office blood pressure recording ≥ 140/90 mmHg and ≤ 160/90 mmHg with good results. Office blood pressure recordings had reduced significantly by 13/7 mmHg at six months.

The feasibility of RDN has been advocated in a wide range of hyper-adrenergic states and anecdotal reports have shown to improve glucose sensitivity, improve quality of life in patients with chronic systolic heart failure, improve sleep-related breathing disorders, improve blood pressure control in chronic renal failure patients, and ameliorate symptoms in patients with heart failure and normal systolic function. However, before implementation, well-designed long-term studies which are rigorously monitored with relevant clinical outcomes as end points are mandated.

Caution should, however, be applied to the widespread application of this procedure, as a large double blind randomized control trial failed to show any benefit. The SIMPLICITY HTN-3 trial was a large, rigorously designed trial which included blinding and a sham treatment in the control arm. It compared renal artery denervation using the Simplicity device in patients with treatment resistant hypertension and systolic blood pressure higher than 160 mmHg with a control arm that included a sham procedure. Five hundred and thirty-five patients were randomly assigned to the two groups that also continued their treatment regimens of three or more antihypertensive drugs at the highest tolerated doses. At six months both groups had demonstrated a significant drop in blood pressure, but there was no statistical difference between the two arms of the study. There were no safety issues with the use of renal denervation. Further trials of renal denervation for hypertension, including those with other devices are ongoing and the future of this type of therapy depends heavily on the outcomes of these trials.

References

Bhatt DL, Kandzari DE, O'Neill WW, et al. for the SYMPLICITY HTN-3 Investigators (2014). A controlled trial of renal denervation for resistant hypertension. New England Journal of Medicine; 370:1393–1401

British Cardiovascular Society. Joint UK Societies Consensus Statement of RenalDenervation for Resistant Hypertension. January 2012. <http://www.bhsoc.org/docs/The-Joint-UK-Societies'-Consensus-on-Renal-Denervation-for-resistant-hypertension.pdf>

DiBona GF. (1994). Neural control of renal function in health and disease. Clinical Autonomic Research; 4:69–94.

Esler MD, Krum H, Sobotka PA, et al. (2010). Renal sympathetic denervation in patients with treatment-resistant hypertension (The Symplicity HTN-2 Trial): a randomised controlled trial. Lancet; 376(9756):1903–9.

Kearney PM, Whelton M, Reynolds K, et al. (2005).Global burden of hypertension: analysis of worldwide data. Lancet; 365(9455): 217–23.

Krum H, Schlaich MP, Bohm M, et al. (2013). Percutaneous renal denervation in patients with treatment-resistant hypertension: final 3-year report of the Symplicity HTN-1 study. Lancet; Nov 6. pii: S0140–6736(13)62192–3

Moser M, Hebert PR (1996). Prevention of disease progression, left ventricular hypertrophy and congestive heart failure in hypertension treatment trials. Journal of the American College of Cardiology; 27(5): 1214–8.

National Institute for Health and Clinical Excellence (2012). Percutaneous transluminal radiofrequency sympathetic denervation of the renal artery for resistant hypertension. NICE IPG 418. January 2012. <http://www.nice.org.uk/nicemedia/live/13340/57923/57923.pdf>.

O'Hagan KP, Thomas GD, Zambraski EJ (1990). Renal denervation decreases blood pressure in DOCA-treated miniature swine with established hypertension. American Journal of Hypertension; 3(1): 62–4.

Pimenta E, Calhoun DA (2012). Resistant hypertension: incidence, prevalence, and prognosis. Circulation; 125(13): 1594–6.

Pimenta E, Oparil S (2012). Renal Sympathetic Denervation for Treatment of Hypertension. Current Treatment Options in Cardiovascular Medicine; Epub ahead of publication.

Symplicity HTN-1 investigators (2011). Catheter-based renal sympathetic denervation for resistant hypertension: durability of blood pressure reduction out to 24 months. Hypertension; 57(5):911–7.

Schlaich MP, Sobotka PA, Krum H, et al. (2009). Renal denervation as a therapeutic approach for hypertension: novel implications for an old concept. Hypertension; 54(6): 1195–201.

Schlaich MP, Schmieder RE, Bakris G, et al. (2013). International Expert Consensus Statement: Percutaneous Transluminal Renal Denervation for the Treatment of Resistant Hypertension; Journal of the American College of Cardiology; 62(22):2031–45.

Chapter 19

Antithrombotic therapy in hypertension

Sunil Nadar

Key points

- Hypertension is associated with a prothrombotic state.
- There is significant platelet activation and endothelial dysfunction seen in hypertensive patients.
- Aspirin has a role in reducing cardiovascular events in patients with multiple cardiovascular risk factors.
- Strict blood pressure control is very important when starting hypertensive patients on aspirin.
- There is no benefit (and perhaps possible harm) in starting hypertensive patients with no cardiovascular risk factors (e.g. young non-diabetic hypertensives) on aspirin.

19.1 Introduction

In hypertension, the vasculature is exposed to high blood pressures. However, hypertension is associated with complications such as myocardial infarction and strokes, which are thrombotic in nature. It is also known that reducing the blood pressure can help prevent these complications. Recently, it has been shown that hypertension is associated with a prothrombotic state. There is significant platelet activation and endothelial dysfunction in hypertension which lead to the prothrombotic state and hence the paradoxical increase in thrombotic complications.

It is therefore postulated that antithrombotic therapy may be beneficial in patients with hypertension with a view to reducing these thrombotic complications, especially as aspirin has been shown to be beneficial in reducing these complications in high-risk individuals. However, the role of antithrombotic agents has not been clearly studied in this setting.

19.2 Clinical trials

Practically all the trials on the use of antiplatelet agents in hypertension involve aspirin as it is the commonest antiplatelet agent used and it is the only agent that has been shown to reduce cardiovascular events in patients at high risk for these events.

The Hypertension Optimal Treatment (HOT) trial was the first study to investigate the use of aspirin as primary prevention in hypertension. In this study, aspirin prevented 1.5 myocardial infarctions per 1000 hypertensive patients per year, which was in addition to the benefit achieved by lowering blood pressure. Indeed, hypertensive patients with an estimated ten-year coronary heart disease (CHD) risk of ≥ 15% will have their cardiovascular risk reduced by 25% using antihypertensive treatment, but the addition of aspirin further reduces major cardiovascular events by 15%. However, in this study, there was no reduction in the number of strokes with aspirin. There was an increase in the number of non-fatal major bleeds but no increase in fatal major bleeds with the use of aspirin as compared to placebo.

A meta-analysis by the Antithrombotic Trialists Collaboration in 2002, looking into the protective role of aspirin in preventing vascular complications, studied more than 100 000 patients with or without elevated blood pressure. They found that aspirin was very effective in preventing complications in 'high-risk' individuals, who included those with previous myocardial infarction or previous cerebrovascular events or other vascular events. The absolute risk reduction (ARR) was 1.1% with a number needed to treat (NNT) of 91. This was mainly due to reduced vascular deaths (NNT = 100), non-fatal myocardial infarctions (NNT = 91), non-fatal stroke (NNT = 200), and the composite outcome measure of major cardiovascular event (ARR = 2.4%, NNT = 42). This analysis also reported that there was no significant difference between the various doses of aspirin that were used (75 mg to 375 mg).

In the subgroup of patients with elevated blood pressure (29 trials, 10 600 patients), antiplatelet therapy significantly reduced major vascular events to a greater extent than the whole analysis (ARR = 4.1%, NNT = 25). All-cause mortality, cardiovascular mortality, non-fatal MI, non-fatal stroke, and haemorrhagic events were not reported in the subgroup of patients with elevated blood pressure.

These data suggest that the absolute benefit for antiplatelet therapy for secondary prevention is greater in patients with elevated blood pressure than in patients with normal blood pressure.

In the subgroup analysis of the Thrombosis Prevention Trial, aspirin reduced coronary events by 20% which was mainly for non-fatal events, and importantly, was significantly greater the lower the systolic blood pressure at entry ($P = 0.0015$). The relative risk at blood pressures of 130 mmHg was 0.55 compared with 0.94 at blood pressures > 145 mmHg. Aspirin also reduced strokes at low but not high blood pressures, the relative risks being 0.41 and 1.42 ($P = 0.006$) respectively. The relative risk of all major cardiovascular events—that is, the sum of coronary heart disease and stroke—was 0.59 at pressures < 130 mmHg, when compared with 1.08 at blood pressures > 145 mmHg ($P = 0.0001$). This analysis therefore suggests that the benefit of low-dose aspirin in primary prevention may occur mainly in those with lower systolic blood pressures, although it is not clear even in these men that the benefit outweighed the potential hazards. In particular, men with higher blood pressures may be exposed to excess risks of bleeding whilst deriving little or no benefit through reductions in coronary heart disease and stroke.

The Antithrombotic trialists in 2009 undertook a meta-analyses of the end result of myocardial infarction, stroke, or vascular death and major bleeds in six primary prevention trials, and 16 secondary prevention trials that compared long-term aspirin versus control. It included 95 000 individuals at low average risk and 17 000 individuals at high average risk respectively. They concluded that in primary prevention without previous disease, aspirin is of uncertain net value as the reduction in occlusive events needs to be weighed against any increase in major bleeds. In the secondary prevention trials, the benefit of aspirin outweighed any potential risk for bleed.

19.3 **Concerns regarding aspirin use**

There are understandably concerns about starting hypertensive patients on antithrombotic therapy in view of the risk of bleeding, given the high pressures that the vessel wall is subjected to. In the HOT study, there was a higher incidence of bleeding in the aspirin group. There was a 1.8% increase of non-fatal, major bleeding events (129 events in patients taking aspirin, compared with 70 in the placebo group) and minor bleeds (156 and 87, respectively). However, there was no increase in the number of fatal bleeding events (seven events in patients taking aspirin, compared with eight in the placebo group). These bleeds were mostly gastrointestinal and nasal, with the increase in bleeding events similar to that seen in other studies of aspirin therapy.

The presence of atrial fibrillation (AF) in hypertensive patients should therefore prompt physicians to control the blood pressure and consider anticoagulation with warfarin, particularly if there are other risk factors present, for example, older age (> 75 years), heart failure, or left ventricular dysfunction. Aspirin has been used as an alternative for thromboprophylaxis in AF and although the data are inconsistent, aspirin is probably useful in younger patients with AF who do not have other cardiovascular risk factors.

Although aspirin is a cheap and widely prescribed drug with a relatively good safety profile, it has many side effects and is often not well tolerated. Many people taking regular aspirin may also develop dyspepsia, the treatment of which will significantly add to the overall cost of therapy. It is also estimated that, aspirin administration may account for as much as one-third of all major gastrointestinal haemorrhage in subjects over 60 years of age, a significant number of which will be fatal. Aspirin can also cause deterioration of renal functions, probably as a result of reduced renal blood flow due to prostaglandin synthesis inhibition.

Another problem with the use of aspirin is the optimal dosage for prophylaxis. Data from the Antiplatelet Trialists Collaboration meta-analyses suggests little difference between the protective effects of medium dose (75–325 mg) and higher doses (500–1500 mg) of aspirin, although these direct comparison were based on only 396 vascular events in three trials. However, higher doses are associated with greater adverse effects.

The use of antithrombotic therapy in hypertensive patients should always be in addition to rigorous and aggressive blood pressure control. The importance of the latter is illustrated by the recent Medical Research Council Thrombosis Prevention Trial, which compared low-intensity oral anticoagulation with warfarin and low-dose aspirin in the primary prevention of ischaemic heart disease in men at increased vascular risk. This study found that the mean blood pressure was highest in those sustaining cerebral haemorrhage, intermediate in those with non-haemorrhagic strokes, and lowest amongst those who did not have strokes.

19.4 **Guidelines**

Recent guidelines by the British Hypertension Society (BHS) recommend the use of 75 mg of aspirin daily for hypertensive patients who have no contraindication to aspirin, in one of the following categories:

(i) *Secondary prevention*: Cardiovascular complications (myocardial infarction, angina, non-haemorrhagic stroke, peripheral vascular disease or atherosclerotic renovascular disease); and

(ii) *Primary prevention*: blood pressure controlled to < 150/90 mmHg and either:

    (a) Age ≥ 50 years and target organ damage (e.g. LVH, renal impairment, or proteinuria); or

    (b) A 10-year CHD risk ≥ 15%; or

    (c) Type 2 diabetes mellitus.

However, some of the risks of aspirin administration—namely, increased incidence of major bleeding events—may possibly outweigh the benefits, especially in low-risk individuals.

Suggested recommendations for the use of antiplatelet drugs in hypertension can be made, according to the following patient categories: (i) high risk requiring secondary prevention, (ii)

Box 19.1 Changes seen in platelets with hypertension

Morphological changes
- Increased volume
- Increased size
- Change in shape
- Increased turnover
- Decreased life span

Biochemical changes
- Increased intracellular free calcium
- Decreased calmodulin levels
- Increased sensitivity to catecholamines
- Higher density of adrenoceptors
- Decreased levels of intracellular catecholamines and serotonin
- Decreased ability to take up monoamines including serotonin
- Decreased intra platelet nitric oxide

Functional changes
- Increased aggregability
- Increased adhesiveness
- Increased spontaneous aggregation

Box 19.2 Practical guidelines for antithrombotic therapy use in the hypertensive patient

- **High-risk hypertensives requiring secondary prevention:** These are the hypertensive patients with a previous heart attack or stroke, or other vascular disease. These patients should receive antithrombotic therapy with aspirin 75 mg daily, in the absence of contraindications.
- **Hypertensives with atrial fibrillation:** Warfarin (INR 2.0–3.0) is recommended in patients who are at high risk for thromboembolism (CHADS2VASC score greater than 2). Aspirin 75–300mg daily can be considered for younger hypertensive patients with AF who have no other risk factors, or along with clopidogrel if warfarin is contraindicated.
- **Hypertensives with other vascular risk factors:** Hypertensives at moderate risk of thrombotic complications may include those with target organ damage (e.g. LVH, renal impairment, or proteinuria), diabetes, hyperlipidaemia, or a strong family history of adverse vascular outcomes or smokers. These patients may benefit more than the low-risk group from aspirin therapy but these additional risk factors need to be identified in a multivariate analysis. The risk–benefit ratio in these patients is still uncertain to recommend widespread prescription of aspirin and individual circumstances should thus be considered.
- **'Lone hypertension':** There is little evidence at present that low-risk individuals with 'lone hypertension', especially those aged under 50 years with no hypertensive target organ damage, will significantly benefit from aspirin therapy and any benefit seen may possibly be outweighed by an increase in bleeding risk. More evidence is needed before aspirin therapy can be recommended for these patients.

NOTE: Blood pressure should be reduced to below 150/90mmHg, and kept well-controlled, with regular clinical surveillance if antithrombotic therapy is to be given.

hypertension with AF (iii) hypertension with other vascular risk factors; and (iv) 'lone' hypertension. 'Lone hypertensive' patients are at lowest risk and there is not much evidence to suggest that they would benefit with antiplatelet therapy and indeed there is the possibility of harm. The 'high-risk' patients are those with previous vascular disease and they would benefit the most with antiplatelet therapy. The other two groups are at moderate risk, and individual decisions have to be made on a patient-to-patient basis as to whether they would benefit from aspirin therapy (Boxes 19.1 and 19.2).

The 2013 Guidelines of the European Cardiac Society recommend that antiplatelet therapy, particularly low-dose aspirin, should be prescribed to controlled hypertensive patients with previous CV events and considered in hypertensive patients with reduced renal function or a high CV risk. Aspirin is not recommended in low- to moderate-risk hypertensive patients in whom absolute benefit and harm are equivalent.

Key references

Antithrombotic Trialists Collaboration (2002). Collaborative meta-analysis of randomised trials of antiplatelet therapy for prevention of death, myocardial infarction, and stroke in high risk patients. *British Medical Journal*; 324: 71–86.

Baigent C, Blackwell L, Collins R, *et al.* (2009) Aspirin in the primary and secondary prevention of vascular disease: collaborative meta-analysis of individual participant data from randomised trials. *Lancet*; 373:1849–60.

British Cardiac Society, British Hyperlipidemia Association, British Hypertension Society, British Diabetic Association (1998). Joint British recommendations on prevention of coronary heart disease in clinical practice. *Heart*; 80(Suppl 2): S1–S29.

Felmeden DC, Lip GY (2005). Antithrombotic therapy in hypertension: a Cochrane Systematic review. *Journal of Human Hypertension*; Mar; 19(3): 185–96.

Hansson L, Zanchetti A, Carruthers SG, *et al.* (1998). Effects of intensive blood-pressure lowering and low-dose aspirin in patients with hypertension: principal results of the Hypertension Optimal Treatment (HOT) randomised trial. HOT Study Group. *Lancet*; 351(9118): 1755–62.

Meade TW, Brennan PJ (2000). Thrombosis Prevention Trial Determination of who may derive most benefit from aspirin in primary prevention: subgroup results from a randomized controlled trial. *British Medical Journal*; 321: 13–17.

The Task Force for the management of arterial hypertension of the European Society of Hypertension (ESH) and of the European Society of Cardiology (ESC) (2013). The 2013 ESH/ESC guidelines on the management of arterial hypertension. *European Heart Journal*; 34:2159–219

Thrombosis Prevention Trial 1998. The Medical Research Council's general Practice Research Framework. Thrombosis prevention trial: randomised trial of low-intensity oral anticoagulation with warfarin and low-dose aspirin in the primary prevention of ischaemic heart disease in men at increased risk. *Lancet*; 351(9098): 233–41.

Part 4

Special conditions

Chapter 20

Hypertension and cardiovascular risk management

Sunil Nadar

Key points

- The objective of treatment of hypertension is to reduce the risk of cardiovascular disease (CVD) and its complications.
- This ensures patients have an increased life expectancy and improved quality of life.
- Treatment is aimed at addressing all risk factors and not the blood pressure readings alone.

20.1 Introduction

Hypertension is an important risk factor for the development of cardiovascular disease (CVD). Both systolic and diastolic blood pressure bear a relationship to cardiovascular morbidity and mortality. Owing to its wide prevalence in the population, hypertension accounts for a significant proportion of annual global death.

The management of patients with hypertension traditionally focused on a target for measured blood pressure values and a variety of drugs to achieve this. The recognition that the majority of patients with hypertension have other co-existing risk factors has moved the emphasis to comprehensive management of cardiovascular risk. The aim of management is to reduce the incidence of fatal and non-fatal cardiovascular events and cerebrovascular events. This is a cost-effective intervention which leads to increased life expectancy and a better quality of life.

20.2 Defining cardiovascular risk

20.2.1 Absolute risk

Hypertension is only one of many factors which contribute to an individual's overall cardiovascular risk. Diabetes, hyperlipidaemia, and obesity are additional risk factors which can be a manifestation of various lifestyle choices—such as high-calorie diet, sedentary lifestyle, and smoking. Multiple co-existing risk factors have a compounding effect in increasing the overall risk.

A number of models have been developed to predict risk.

1. The WHO/ISH risk prediction charts measure ten-year risk of a fatal or non-fatal myocardial infarction or stroke based on age, sex, blood pressure, smoking status, total blood cholesterol, and presence or absence of diabetes mellitus. They contain a number of charts appropriate to the different global areas.

2. The Joint British Societies' CVD risk prediction estimates the risk of developing CVD—coronary heart disease (CHD) and stroke over ten years. The factors taken into consideration are age, sex, smoking status, systolic blood pressure, and the ratio of total cholesterol to HDL cholesterol.

3. Framingham Risk Equations—these are useful in estimating the ten-year risk of developing heart failure, coronary disease, or stroke. The limitations of this estimate are that it consists of data from predominantly white middle-class people from the United States. They also do not account for obesity and lifestyle choices.

These and other risk models have been developed to help the decision-making process with regards treatment for hypertension and other co-existing risk factors. None of these, however, account for ethnicity which can significantly increase the risk, especially in the South Asian population.

20.2.2 Relative risk

Population-based studies have shown a consistent relationship between blood pressure recordings and the development of vascular events in the future. Treating high blood pressure reduces the risk but the exact relationship between the degree of reduction in risk and the extent to which the blood pressure is reduced remains unclear.

All models of quantifying risk aim to be simple and easy to use in order to be widely applicable. Their limitations include being unable to incorporate the length of time that various risks have been present into calculations and they attribute limited significance to variables such as exercise. Especially in the younger age group, patients may have a number of major risk factors and be at significantly high relative risk but might still appear to have a small absolute risk. The converse is also true; in older age groups the presence of a risk factor can appear to confer a high absolute risk on development although the individual's risk relative to their peers might not be significantly higher. This is particularly relevant to younger patients who, in the absence of appropriate treatment, might be exposed to significant risk over a prolonged period of time causing irreversible damage.

20.3 Triggers for treating risk factors

In the presence of significant relative risk for adverse events from cardiovascular disease, treatment helps in reducing events. Risk factors include pre-existing cardiovascular disease, diabetes mellitus, CVD risk > 20% over ten years, a high total cholesterol or elevated cholesterol-to-HDL ratio and the presence of systolic blood pressure greater than 160 mmHg or a diastolic greater than 100 mmHg. With evidence of end-organ damage such as left ventricular hypertrophy (LVH), elevated serum creatinine, microalbuminuria, or reduced estimated glomerular filtration rate (eGFR), the overall risk is elevated even at lower levels of blood pressure.

20.4 Managing risk factors that affect cardiovascular disease

- Decisions to treat are based on relative risks.
- Treatment includes modifications to lifestyle alongside drug therapy.
- Treatment is prioritized to the greatest risk factors.
- Therapy aims to maximize benefit while minimizing the adverse effects.

A number of risk factors are inherent in an individual and are not modifiable. These include age, male sex, family history, and ethnicity. Modifiable risk factors can be favourably altered

	Blood pressure (mmHg)				
Other risk factors OD or disease	Normal SBP 120–129 or DBP 80–84	High normal SBP 130–139 or DBP 85–89	Grade 1 HT SBP 140–159 or DBP 90–99	Grade 2 HT SBP 140–159 or DBP 90–99	Grade 3 HT SBP ≥ 180 DBP ≥ 110
No other risk factors	No BP intervention	No BP intervention	Lifestyle changes for several months then drug treatment if BP uncontrolled	Lifestyle changes for several weeks then drug treatment if BP uncontrolled	Lifestyle changes + Immediate drug treatment
1–2 risk factors	Lifestyle changes	Lifestyle changes	Lifestyle changes for several weeks then drug treatment if BP uncontrolled	Lifestyle changes for several weeks then drug treatment if BP uncontrolled	Lifestyle changes + Immediate drug treatment
≥3 risk factors, Ms or OD	Lifestyle changes	Lifestyle changes and consider drug treatment	Lifestyle changes + Drug treatment	Lifestyle changes + Drug treatment	Lifestyle changes + Immediate drug treatment
Diabetes	Lifestyle changes	Lifestyle changes + Drug treatment	Lifestyle changes + Drug treatment	Lifestyle changes + Drug treatment	Lifestyle changes + Immediate drug treatment
Established CV or renal disease	Lifestyle changes + Immediate drug treatment	Lifestyle changes + Immediate drug treatment	Lifestyle changes + Immediate drug treatment	Lifestyle changes + Immediate drug treatment	Lifestyle changes + Immediate drug treatment

Figure 20.1 European Society of Hypertension (ESH) guidelines on the initiation of treatment based on cardiovascular risk

Key: OD = Organ damage, CV = Cardiovascular, MS = Metabolic syndrome. Figure 8.1 is reproduced from Mancia G, De Backer G, Dominiczak A, et al. (2007), Guidelines for the management of arterial hypertension: The Task Force for the Management of Arterial Hypertension of the European Society of Hypertension (ESH) and of the European Society of Cardiology (ESC). *Eur. Heart J.*, **28**: 1462.-536, with permission from Oxford University Press.

either by drug therapy or behavioural change. Figure 20.1 presents the views of the European Society of Hypertension on the management strategy of hypertensive patients based on their cardiovascular risk.

20.5 **Non-drug interventions**

Lifestyle modification has a role to play in reducing cardiovascular risk. Many of these interventions can help lower blood pressure or delay the progression to conditions such as diabetes. These measures are generally helpful but not proven to prevent complications from CVD and compliance in the long term is usually poor.

Dietary interventions are aimed at the following:

- Reducing intake of total calories, salt, and fat in the daily diet. This helps in a number of ways. Reducing the dietary sodium intake (salt) has shown to reduce blood pressure. Reduced calorie intake allows weight reduction in overweight individuals which has a beneficial effect on blood pressure.

- Increasing the intake of fruit and vegetables. Increases in daily potassium intake and a diet high in fruit and vegetables have been shown to reduce the blood pressure.

- Regular exercise. Regular physical activity reduces blood pressure and body fat. Additional benefits such as improved insulin sensitivity and an increase in HDL cholesterol are also seen. Changes to a sedentary lifestyle are important in maintaining an ideal body weight.

- Moderation of alcohol consumption. Studies have consistently shown that individuals who consume small or moderate amounts of alcohol have a lower cardiovascular mortality than non-drinkers. Heavy drinking is associated with significant morbidity.

20.5.1 **Smoking cessation**

Smoking causes rise of blood pressure and heart rate. Stopping smoking may not directly lower blood pressure but it significantly reduces the cardiovascular risk. Smoking cessation should be offered as part of a structured programme including counseling and nicotine replacement therapy.

20.6 **Drug treatments aimed at reducing risk**

The decision to treat other risk factors is based on the added risk in each hypertensive individual. Treatment strategies include the following.

20.6.1 **Antiplatelet therapy**

The benefits and risks of aspirin therapy in hypertensive patients has been shown in the Hypertension Optimal Treatment (HOT) study. Overall, the study showed a 15% reduction in major cardiovascular events, and a 36% reduction in acute myocardial infarction, with no effect on stroke and no increased risk of intracerebral haemorrhage but an associated 65% increased risk of major haemorrhagic events. Patients with serum creatinine > 115 μmol/L (>1.3 mg/dL), and those with a higher cardiovascular risk at baseline had a favourable risk–benefit balance. In hypertensives at lower baseline risk the harm of aspirin counterbalanced the benefits.

The European, British, and American guidelines recommend that patients with pre-existing vascular disease would be candidates for long-term treatment with low-dose aspirin. Aspirin significantly reduces the risk of recurrent vascular events though the risk of extracranial bleeds is almost doubled. Patients who have had previous bleeding problems associated with aspirin could be considered for treatment with clopidogrel instead. Because of the risk of bleeding with aspirin a clear benefit with anti-platelet treatment is seen only in patients who have a 15–20% 10-year cardiovascular risk. To minimize the risk of haemorrhagic stroke, aspirin should only be started once good blood pressure control has been achieved. This topic is discussed in greater detail in Chapter 17 of this book.

20.6.2 **Lipid-lowering agents**

Several studies have demonstrated the benefit of statins in lowering cardiovascular events. In the Heart Protection Study, administration of simvastatin to patients with established cardiovascular disease led to a marked reduction in cardiac and cerebrovascular events compared to placebo. Hypertensives accounted for around 41% of the entire cohort and this effect was seen in this subgroup as well, irrespective of the type of antihypertensive agent used. Similar results were obtained with pravastatin in the Pravastatin in Elderly Individuals at Risk of Vascular Disease (PROSPER) study, where 62% of trial subjects were hypertensive. Atorvastatin has also been shown to be effective in preventing cardiovascular disease in the Anglo Scandinavian Cardiac Outcomes Trial (ASCOT). Most guidelines therefore suggest that patients up to the age of at least 80 years who have an established cardiovascular disease or long-term (at least ten years) diabetes should receive a statin. In all these patients the goal for total and LDL serum cholesterol should be set at respectively < 4.5 mmol/L (175 mg/dl) and < 2.5 mmol/L (100 mg/dL), and lower goals may also be considered, i.e. < 4.0 and < 2 mmol/L (155 and 80 mg/dL).

Two trials, the Antihypertensive and Lipid-Lowering Treatment to Prevent Heart Attack Trial (ALLHAT) and ASCOT, have evaluated the benefits associated with the use of statins (pravastatin and atorvastatin, respectively) specifically among patients with hypertension. Whilst ALLHAT did not demonstrate any benefit with pravastatin in hypertensive patients with cardiovascular disease, ASCOT demonstrated a substantial benefit to the group that was given atorvastatin. The beneficial effect seen in the ASCOT trial as compared to the lack of benefit reported in ALLHAT may depend on the greater relative difference in total and LDL cholesterol achieved among the actively treated versus the control group.

The European Society of Hypertension (ESH) and the European Society of Cardiology (ESC), in their guidelines suggest that statin therapy should be considered in hypertensive patients aged less than 80 years who have an estimated ten-year risk of cardiovascular disease of 20% or more or of cardiovascular death of 5% or more. Target levels should be a serum total and LDL cholesterol of respectively < 5mmol/L (190 mg/dL) and < 3 mmol/L (115 mg/dL). The majority of patients will reach these targets using a statin at appropriate doses in combination with non-pharmacological measures. For patients who do not reach targets or whose HDL cholesterol or triglyceride levels remain abnormal (e.g. < 1.0 mmol/L, > 2.3 mmol/L, respectively), addition of ezetimibe or other therapies as well as referral to a specialist service may be indicated.

The Joint British Societies' guidelines also suggest that treatment with statin should aim to achieve total cholesterol of 5.0 mmol/L or less (or a 25% reduction in total cholesterol), and LDL cholesterol of 3.0 mmol/L or less (or a 30% reduction in LDL cholesterol).

20.6.3 **Control of blood sugars**

The aim of management of blood sugars is early detection with the goal to prevent progression to diabetes. Diabetes and impaired glucose tolerance are significant risk factors for the development of cardiovascular disease. Hypertension is common with type 2 diabetes and diabetic hypertensive patients have a marked increase in total cardiovascular risk. Similarly, hypertension is associated with an increased risk of developing type 2 diabetes. Strict control of blood sugars is important in these patients. In the United Kingdom Prospective Diabetes Study (UKPDS), hypertensive patients with type 2 diabetes benefited from intensive blood glucose control mainly in terms of microvascular complications. Other studies have shown protection against macrovascular complications as well with strict glycaemic control.

According to guidelines for the management of diabetes the treatment goals are set to ≤ 6.0 mmol/L (108 mg/dL) for plasma preprandial glucose concentrations (average of several measurements), and at less than 6.5% for glycated haemoglobin. The treatment of diabetic hypertensive patients is discussed in detail in Chapter 26.

20.7 Summary

In conclusion, the management of hypertension has evolved. It is not just about controlling the blood pressure and treating blood pressure values. It includes treating the overall cardio-vascular risk in an individual. Recent guidelines by the British Hypertension Society and the American and European societies of hypertension have recommended treatment of these patients with lipid-lowering and antiplatelet agents in order to reduce overall cardiovascular risk. Thus, treating a hypertensive individual entails a comprehensive and holistic cardiovascular risk management strategy.

Key references

JBS (2005). Joint British Societies' guidelines on prevention of cardiovascular disease in clinical practice. *Heart;* 91(Suppl V): v1–v52.

Pignone M, Mulrow CD (2001). Using cardiovascular risk profiles to individualize hypertensive treatment. *British Medical Journal;* 322: 1164–6.

NICE (2007). Clinical guideline 34-Hypertension: management of hypertension in adults in primary care. NICE Publications, London. <http://www.nice.org.uk>

<http://www.nice.org.uk/nicemedia/pdf/CG034NICEguideline.doc>

Padwal R, Strauss S, McAlister FA, et al. (2001). Cardiovascular risk factors and their effects on the decision to treat hypertension: evidence based review. *British Medical Journal;* 322: 977–80.

World Health Organization (2007). Prevention of Cardiovascular Disease—Pocket Guidelines for Assessment and Management of Cardiovascular Risk. Geneva: WHO.

The Task Force for the management of arterial hypertension of the European Society of Hypertension (ESH) and of the European Society of Cardiology (ESC) (2013). 2013 ESH/ESC Guidelines for the management of arterial hypertension. *European Heart Journal;* 34, 2159–219.

Chapter 21

Guidelines on the pharmacological management of hypertension

Gregory YH Lip and Sunil Nadar

Key points

- British and European guidelines have classified systolic blood pressure of 130–139 mmHg as 'high normal' (the American guidelines call this 'prehypertension') and do not recommend pharmacological treatment but strict lifestyle modification for this group.
- Different classes of antihypertensive agents are recommended depending on comorbidities and risk factors.
- Treatment is holistic and should encompass cardiovascular risk management in addition to blood pressure management.
- Latest guidelines do not recommend a lower target systolic blood pressure for diabetics.

143

21.1 Introduction

Given the rapid advances in management of patients with hypertension, guidelines on appropriate investigations and treatments (both pharmacological and non-pharmacological) have regularly been issued by learned bodies to inform the medical community on optimal approach to such patients.

The commonest guidelines in clinical use are those from the British Hypertension Society (BHS), the Joint National Committee (JNC) on Prevention, Detection, Evaluation, and Treatment of High Blood Pressure and the European Society of Hypertension (ESH) guidelines. Other guidelines have been issued by the World Health Organization (WHO) along with the International Society of hypertension (ISH) and in the United Kingdom, we also have the guidelines issued by the National Institute for Health and Care Excellence (NICE), which issues evidence-based management guidelines based on cost-effectiveness, and more recently has issued joint guidelines with the BHS.

For this chapter, we will mainly discuss the BHS/NICE, European guidelines (2013), and the JNC-8 guidelines.

All modern hypertension guidelines are fairly similar in the approach tof cardiovascular risk assessment as hypertension is no longer a disease in isolation but part of cardiovascular risk continuum. The initial part of the published guidelines usually include guidance on how to measure blood pressure accurately, assessment methods for cardiovascular risk in these patients, and methods of investigating hypertensive patients. The documents then give guidance on non-pharmacological and pharmacological treatment and management of special conditions such as hypertension in pregnancy, malignant hypertension, renal damage, etc.

All of the areas covered by the guideline documents have been covered in other chapters of this book. Thus, we will concentrate on the treatment algorithms that have been recommended in various guidelines.

Table 21.1 Blood pressure thresholds for treatment		
Blood pressure	**Comment**	**Recommendation**
< 130/85		Reassess in five years
130–139/85–89		Reassess yearly but strict lifestyle modification
140–159/90–99	No TOD, no cardiovascular complications, no diabetes, no renal failure and ten-year CVD risk < 20%	Observe, reassess CVD risk yearly, lifestyle modification
140–159/90–99	TOD or cardiovascular complications or diabetes or renal failure or ten-year CVD risk > 20%	Treat pharmacologically
> 160/100		Treat pharmacologically

TOD: target organ damage, CVD: cardiovascular disease.

21.2 British Hypertension Society/NICE guidelines

The BHS-IV guidelines do not use the term 'prehypertension'. Instead they use the term 'high normal' blood pressure. In the non-diabetic, no pharmacological treatment is recommended for the normal and high normal individual (SBP < 139 mmHg and DBP < 89 mmHg). For this group yearly monitoring and strict lifestyle modification education is recommended.

Pharmacological treatment is advised in all the other groups on top of lifestyle modification (Table 21.1). The various drugs that can be used are summarized in Table 21.2 with the scenarios where one drug would be preferred over the other.

In patients younger than 80 years of age, a target of 140/90 mmHg is recommended on treatment. For patients aged over 80 years, the target on treatment should be 150/90 mmHg. For patients aged less than 40 years with stage 1 hypertension, and no evidence of target organ

Table 21.2 Compelling and possible indications for the major classes of drugs		
	Compelling indication	**Possible indication**
Thiazide/Thiazide-like diuretics	Elderly, heart failure, isolated systolic hypertension	
Calcium-channel blockers	Elderly, isolated systolic hypertension	Elderly, ischaemic heart disease (rate limiting non-dihydropyridine agents)
Beta blockers	Ischaemic heart disease	Heart failure (with caution, under supervision)
ACE inhibitors	Heart failure, post myocardial infarction, type i diabetic nephropathy, stroke prevention	Chronic renal disease, type 2 diabetic nephropathy, proteinuric renal disease
Angiotensin receptor blockers	ACE inhibitor intolerance, type 2 diabetic nephropathy, presence of left ventricular hypertrophy	Left ventricular dysfunction post-myocardial infarction
Alpha blockers	Benign prostatic hypertrophy Benign prostatic hypertrophy	

damage, cardiovascular disease, renal disease, or diabetes, consider seeking specialist evaluation of secondary causes of hypertension and a more detailed assessment of potential target organ damage. This is because ten-year cardiovascular risk assessments can underestimate the lifetime risk of cardiovascular events in these people.

Figure 21.1 gives the recommended treatment algorithm in the joint BHS/NICE guidelines issued in 2011. In brief, step 1 is monotherapy with either an ACE inhibitor or an angiotensin receptor blocker (ARB) for patients with low renin states such as young patients or non-Afro-Caribbean patients. For older patients or patients of Afro-Caribbean origin, a calcium-channel blocker is recommended. For patients who are unable to tolerate a calcium-channel blocker due to oedema of if there are heart failure-like symptoms, a thiazide like diruetic (chlortalidone or indapamide) can be started rather than the conventional thiazide diuretic.

Beta blockers are not a preferred initial therapy for hypertension.

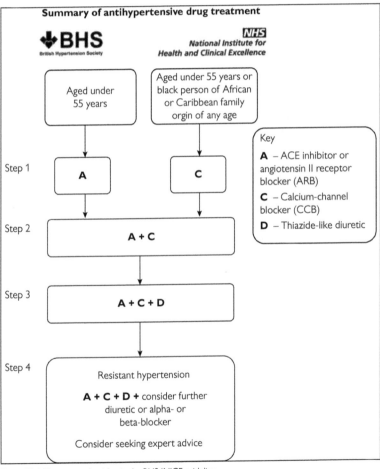

Figure 21.1 Treatment algorithm in the BHS/NICE guideline

National Institute for Health and Clinical Excellence (2006) CG34 Hypertension: clinical management of primary hypertension in adults. Manchester: NICE. Available from http://www.nice.org.uk/guidance/CG34 Reproduced with permission

However, they may be considered in younger people, particularly in those with an intolerance or contraindication to ACE inhibitors and angiotensin II receptor antagonists **or** women of child-bearing potential **or** people with evidence of increased sympathetic drive. If, however, a second-line agent has to be added to a beta blocker, a calcium-channel blocker rather than a thiazide diuretic is recommended to decrease the chance of developing diabetes.

Step 2 would be adding a second drug, for example, an ACE inhibitor to either the calcium-channel blocker or the diuretic. A combination of an ACE inhibitor and ARB should be avoided. Step 3 would be adding all three and step 4 would be adding a different agent such as a beta blocker, an alpha blocker, or another diuretic. At that stage, it is recommended to refer to a specialist, if blood pressure remains uncontrolled.

Other factors mentioned in the guidelines are adjunctive agents used to reduce cardiovascular risk. For example, it is recommended that patients with established cardiovascular disease or at high risk according to the Joint British Societies' cardiovascular disease risk chart computer programme or cardiovascular disease risk chart should be considered for aspirin and statin therapy as follows:

- For primary prevention: aspirin 75 mg is recommended for hypertensive patients aged 50 years or more who have satisfactory control over their blood pressure and either target organ damage, diabetes, or cardiovascular disease risk > 20%.

- For primary prevention: statin therapy is indicated when the ten-year cardiovascular disease risk is > 20%.

- For secondary prevention: statin therapy and aspirin therapy are indicated when there is evidence of cardiovascular disease, that is, angina/myocardial infarction, stroke, transient ischaemic attack, peripheral vascular disease, etc.

21.3 The joint EHS/ESC guidelines 2013

In the EHS/ESC guidelines, the definitions and classification of hypertension are as shown in Table 21.3.

The real threshold for defining "hypertension" is defined as being high or low based on the total CV risk of each individual.

These guidelines make reference to the Systematic COronary Risk Evaluation (SCORES) risk score, which was first proposed in the 2003 European Guidelines on Cardiovascular

Table 21.3 Definitions and classifications of blood pressure (BP) levels (mmHg)			
Category	Systolic		Diastolic
Optimal	< 120	and	< 80
Normal	120–129	and/or	80–84
High normal	130–139	and/or	85–89
Grade 1 hypertension	140–159	and/or	90–99
Grade 2 hypertension	160–179	and/or	100–109
Grade 3 hypertension	≥ 180	and/or	≥ 110
Isolated systolic hypertension	≥ 140	and	< 90

Isolated systolic hypertension should be graded (1, 2, 3) according to systolic blood pressure values in the ranges indicated, providede that diastolic values are < 90 mmHg.

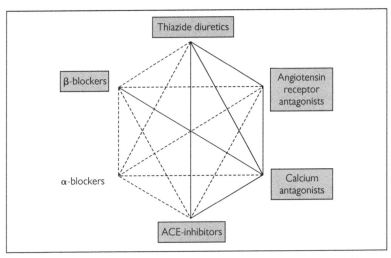

Figure 21.2 Recommended combinations of antihypertensive therapy as recommended by the European Society of Hypertension

The preferred combinations in the general hypertensive population are represented as thick lines. The frames indicate classes of agents proven to be beneficial in controlled intervention trials.

Authors/Task Force Members et al, Eur Heart J 2007 28:1462–1536.

Disease Prevention in Clinical Practice. These CV mortality risk scores were derived from data from over 200 000 individuals from 11 European countries, who were followed up for approximately 13 years for CV death. In this schema, the corresponding SCORE colour charts provide ten-year risk for individuals aged 40–65 years, in relation to sex, cholesterol, SBP, and smoking status—and in the guideline, risk charts for 'high-risk' and 'low-risk' countries are provided. In these guidelines, the benefits of blood pressure lowering due to the impact on measured blood pressure *per se* are stressed and not which drug or drug combination is used or in which order they should be introduced. Combinations recommended are shown in Figure 21.2.

The individual patient's treatment is in relation to blood pressure lowering and to drug side effects, the specific cardiovascular risk profile of the patient, and the presence of target organ damage concomitant disease factors, etc.—as shown in the Table 21.4 and Figure 21.3. The guidelines do highlight some conditions favouring the use of some antihypertensive drugs over others.

21.4 JNC-7 and 8 guidelines

The JNC guidelines are fairly similar to the BHS-IV. As mentioned, one of the main differences is the classification of 'prehypertension' as a separate entity. The new JNC-8 guidelines do not deal much with the diagnosis and investigations of hypertension, but comment mainly on the management.

The difference with the NICE/BHS guidelines is the age cut off. As per the JNC guidelines, for patients aged 60 years and above (as opposed to 80 years as per the NICE/BHS guidelines), pharmacologic treatment should be started if BP is greater than 150/90 mmHg and treated to a target of less than 150/90 mmHg. For adult patients aged less than 60 years, and

Table 21.4 Choice of antihypertensive agent depending on the presence of target organ damage or comorbidity

Subclinical organ damage	
LVH	
Asymptomatic atherosclerosis	ACEL, CA, ARB
	CA, ACEI
Microalbuminuria	ACEL ARB
Renal dysfunction	ACEL ARB
Clinical event	
Previous stroke	any BP lowering agent BB ACEL, ARBBB, CA diureties,
Previous MI	BB, ACEI, ARB, anti-aldosterone agents
Angina pectoris	
Heart failure	
Atrial fibrillation	
Recurrent	ARB, ACEI
Permanent	BB, non-dihydropiridine CA
Tachyarrhythmias	BB
ESRD/proteinuria	ACEI ARB loop diuretics
Peripheral artery disease	CA
LV dysfunction	ACEI
Condition	
ISH (elderly)	diuretics CA
Metabolic syndrome	ACEL, ARB, CA
Diabetes mellitus	ACEL, ARB,
Pregnancy	CA methyldopa, BB
Black people	BB
Glaucoma	ARB
ACEI-induced cough	

LVH = left ventricular hypertrophy; ISH = Isolated systolic hypertension; ESRD = renal failure; ACEI = ACE-inhibitors; ARB = angiotensin receptor antagonists; CA = calcium antagonists; BB = beta blockers.

those with chronic renal failure or diabetes, treatment should be started at BP greater than 140/90 mmHg and treated to a goal of less than 140/90 mmHg.

The rest of the treatment algorithm is fairly similar to the other guidelines, in terms of starting on either a thiazide diuretic, or calcium-channel blocker or ACE inhibitor or ARB, and then adding another agent in the next stage and so on.

21.5 Comparison with the other guidelines

In general most of the recent guidelines are similar. Table 21.5 highlights some of the major differences

1) The age cut off between different targets is different. The European and British guidelines recommend a higher treatment target (150/90 mmHg) for patients that are aged 80 and above, whilst the JNC-8 uses 60 years as a cut off.

2) For diabetics, the European guidelines use 140/85 mmHg as the target, whilst the JNC use 140/90 mmHg as target

Other risk factors, asymptomatic organ damage or disease	Blood pressure (mmHg)			
	High normal SBP 130–139 or DBP 85–39	Grade 1 HT SBP 140–159 or DBP 90–99	Grade 2 HT SBP 160–179 or DBP 100–109	Grade 3 HT SBP ≥180 or DBP ≥110
No other RF		Low risk	Moderate risk	High risk
1–2 RF	Low risk	Moderate risk	Moderate to high risk	High risk
≥3 RF	Low to Moderate risk	Moderate to high risk	High risk	High risk
OD, CND stage 3 or diabetes	Moderate to high risk	High risk	High risk	High to very high risk
Symptomatic CVD, CND stage ≥ 4 or diabetes with 0D/RFs	Very high risk	Very high risk	Very high risk	Very high risk

Figure 21.3 Guidelines on management depending on cardiovascular risk

BP = blood pressure; CKD = chronic kidney disease; CV = cardiovascular; CVD = cardiovascular disease; DBP = diastolic blood pressure, HT = hypertension, OD = organ damage; RF = risk factor; SBP = systolic blood pressure. Authors/Task Force Members et al, *Eur Heart J* 2007 28:1462–1536.

Table 21.5 Comparison of the different guidelines			
Guideline	Population	Goal BP (mmHg)	Initial drug treatment options
JNC-8	General > 60yrs	< 150/90	Non-black: thiazide type diuretic, ACEI,ARB or CCB
	General < 60 yrs	< 140/90	Black: thiazide like diuretic or CCB
	Diabetes	< 140/90	
	CKD	< 140/90	ACEI or ARB
ESH/ESC	General non elderly	< 140/90	Diuretic, beta blocker, CCB, ACEI or ARB
	General elderly < 80	< 150/90	
	General > 80	< 150/90	
	Diabetes	< 140/85	ACEI or ARB
	CKD no proteinuria	< 140/90	ACEI or ARB
	CKD with proteinuria	130/90	
NICE	General < 80	140/90	< 55yrs ACEI or ARB; > 55 or black- CCB
	General > 80	< 150/90	

3) The ESH guidelines have a lower target of 130/80 mmHg for patients with renal failure and proteinuria, whilst the JNC-8 do not make this differentiation within the renal failure group.

Key references

James PA, Oparil S, Carter BL, et al. (2014) Evidence-Based Guideline for the Management of High Blood Pressure in Adults: Report From the Panel Members Appointed to the Eighth Joint National Committee (JNC 8)

Journal of the American Medical Association; 311(5):507–20.

Hypertension: Clinical management of primary hypertension in adults. The NICE guidelines. <http://publications.nice.org.uk/hypertension-cg127>

The Task Force for the management of arterial hypertension of the European Society of Hypertension (ESH) and of the European Society of Cardiology (ESC) (2013). 2013 ESH/ESC Guidelines for themanagement of arterial hypertension. *Journal of Hypertension*; 31:1281–357.

Chapter 22

Hypertension in pregnancy

VJ Karthikeyan

Key points

- Hypertension is one of the commonest medical problems seen during pregnancy.
- Hypertension during pregnancy may be pre-existing or may develop during pregnancy when it is called gestational hypertension or pregnancy-induced hypertension.
- Hypertensive disorders of pregnancy have a high rate of recurrence during subsequent pregnancies.
- Pharmacological treatment has not been shown conclusively to reduce neonatal complications.
- Eclampsia and pre-eclampsia are considered medical emergencies and should be carefully monitored and treated.

22.1 Introduction

Hypertension is the most common medical condition that occurs in pregnancy, is a leading cause of maternal mortality, and has other serious effects on pregnancy outcomes. It occurs in around 5% of all pregnancies. However, this covers a wide range of conditions that carry different implications for pregnancy outcome and require different management strategies. Hypertension in pregnancy affects both the mother and the foetus, and can lead to severe maternal and foetal morbidity and mortality if not diagnosed and treated early.

Hypertensive diseases of pregnancy including eclampsia and pre-eclampsia are the second major cause of maternal and foetal mortality in the United Kingdom (mortality rate around 2%). Eclampsia is responsible for one-sixth of all maternal deaths.

22.2 Classification of hypertension in pregnancy

Hypertensive disorders in pregnancy are classified into four categories according to the Working Group Report on Hypertension in Pregnancy as chronic hypertension, pre-eclampsia-eclampsia, pre-eclampsia superimposed upon chronic hypertension, and gestational hypertension (Table 22.1).

Chronic hypertension is hypertension (blood pressure ≥ 140 mmHg systolic and/ or ≥ 90 mmHg diastolic) that is present and observable before pregnancy or diagnosed before the 20th week of gestation as well as that diagnosed for the first time during pregnancy and that persists into the post-partum period.

Pre-eclampsia and eclampsia are pregnancy-specific syndromes that usually occurs after 20 weeks' gestation, or earlier in trophoblastic diseases (hydatidiform mole or hydrops). The increased blood pressure is accompanied by proteinuria in this syndrome.

Table 22.1 Hypertensive disorders in pregnancy

Findings	Chronic hypertension	Gestational hypertension	Pre-eclampsia or eclampsia
Time of onset of hypertension	< 20 weeks of gestation	After mid-pregnancy	≥ 20 weeks of gestation
Proteinuria	Absent	Absent	Present
Haemoconcentration	Absent	Absent	Present
Thrombocytopaenia	Absent	Absent	Present
Hepatic dysfunction	Absent	Absent	Present
Serum creatinine > 1.2 mg/dL	Absent	Absent	Present
Raised serum uric acid	Absent	Absent	Present
Clinical symptoms	Absent	Absent	Present

Pre-eclampsia is a syndrome characterized by hypertension, proteinuria, and symptoms of headache, visual changes, epigastric or right upper quadrant pain, and dyspnoea. Several factors have been identified to be associated with an increased risk of pre-eclampsia such as age, parity, previous pre-eclampsia, family history, multiple pregnancy, pre-existing medical conditions (insulin dependent diabetes mellitus [IDDM]), obesity and insulin resistance, chronic hypertension, renal disease, autoimmune disease, anti-phospholipid syndrome, rheumatic disease), smoking, increased body mass index (BMI), raised blood pressure, and proteinuria. In addition, couple-related factors including limited sperm exposure, primipaternity, pregnancies after donor insemination/oocyte/embryo donation have been found to play an important role too.

Eclampsia is the occurrence of seizures in a woman with pre-eclampsia that cannot be attributed to other causes.

Gestational hypertension or pregnancy-induced hypertension (PIH) occurs with a blood pressure > 140/90 mmHg in a woman who was normotensive before 20 weeks' gestation. Severe gestational hypertension is a condition of sustained elevation in blood pressure of > 160/110 mmHg for six hours. Blood pressure normalizes in the post-partum period usually within ten days. Patients may experience headache, blurred vision, and abdominal pain and are noted to have abnormal lab tests, including low platelet counts and abnormal liver function tests.

Pre-eclampsia may occur in women with chronic hypertension, with a much worse prognosis than with either condition alone. Superimposed pre-eclampsia is difficult to distinguish from worsening chronic hypertension, with possible findings that include new onset proteinuria in women with hypertension and no proteinuria in early pregnancy (< 20 weeks' gestation), sudden increase in proteinuria or blood pressure in a woman with previously well controlled hypertension, thrombocytopenia (< 100 000 platelets/mm^3), or abnormal elevation in liver enzymes (alanine aminotransferase or aspartate aminotransferase).

22.3 **Measurement of blood pressure**

Measurement of diastolic blood pressure during pregnancy has been a topic of debate. Suffice it to mention that the National High Blood Pressure Education Program Working Group on High Blood Pressure in Pregnancy (NHBPEP) recommends the use of Korotkoff phase V.

> **Box 22.1** Tests for pre-eclamapsia
>
> Clinical tests
> - Average second trimester mean arterial pressure (MAP) ≥ 90 mmHg
> - Angiotensin infusion test
> - Uterine artery Doppler waveforms
> - Laboratory tests
> - Urinary calcium
> - Urine kallikrein to creatinine ratio
> - Plasma fibronectin
> - Serum inhibin
> - Serum alpha foeto protein (AFP)/ HCG (human chorionic gonadotrophin)
> - Serum urate
> - Hematocrit
> - Antithrombin III
> - Plasminogen activator inhibitors (1 and 2)

22.4 **Pathophysiology**

Pre-eclampsia is caused by the presence of the placenta or the maternal response to placentation. Poor placentation is a strong predisposing factor that leads to the maternal syndrome, the extent of which is related to the inflammatory signals (dependent on foetal genes) as well as the nature of the maternal responses (dependent on maternal genes).

Two diverse theories, vascular (ischaemia-reperfusion resulting in oxidative stress and vascular disease) and immune (maternal–paternal immune maladaptation, i.e. a maternal alloimmune reaction triggered by a rejection of foetal allograft) are hypothesized to be responsible for pre-eclampsia. The aetio-pathophysiology of pre-eclampsia is complex and involves diverse factors such as genetic predisposition, disturbances in the renin–angiotensin–aldosterone axis, dysfunction of the maternal endothelium, maternal coagulopathies, cytokines, growth factors, and so on.

Although various clinical and laboratory tests (Box 22.1) are currently used to predict the risk of women developing pre-eclampsia, no test reliably predicts it. The importance of clinical history cannot be overemphasized here.

22.5 **Management of hypertension in pregnancy**

22.5.1 **Prevention of pre-eclampsia**

Several measures such as calcium supplementation, low-dose aspirin, and fish oils have been suggested to help prevent pre-eclampsia and have had varied results.

22.5.2 **Monitoring of patients with hypertension during pregnancy**

Baseline laboratory investigations (hematocrit, hemoglobin concentration, platelet count, and serum creatinine and uric acid levels) early during gestation, with monitoring of levels are particularly useful in the early diagnosis of pre-eclampsia.

Proteinuria of 1+ by routine urinalysis is an indication for a 24-hour collection for protein and creatinine estimation to determine accuracy of collection and estimation of creatinine clearance. Accurate dating (with ultrasonographic methods, if required) and assessment of foetal growth in high-risk patients is important, as is a baseline ultrasound scan at 25–28 weeks' gestation to evaluate foetal growth.

In women presenting with hypertension after mid-pregnancy, laboratory tests are recommended, with bi-weekly monitoring to distinguish pre-eclampsia from chronic and transient hypertension as well as to assess disease progression and severity. One or more abnormalities may be present in women with pre-eclampsia despite relatively minimal blood pressure elevations. A life-threatening abnormality such as coagulopathy or abnormal hepatic and/or renal function may necessitate termination of pregnancy despite only mild hypertension.

Treatment of hypertension (particularly systolic hypertension) promptly and effectively is of utmost importance in the prevention of complications such as haemorrhagic stroke. Iatrogenic hypertension is best avoided by abandoning the use of ergometrine in the routine management of third-stage of labour.

22.5.3 **Chronic hypertension in pregnancy**

Women with hypertension require a full assessment of the severity of hypertension and advice on lifestyle changes (restriction of daily activities, refraining from vigorous exercise, restriction of daily sodium intake, stopping smoking and alcohol intake). Discontinuation of drugs known to be harmful to the foetus is particularly important, with a switch to safer alternatives. Those with target organ damage should be warned regarding the higher risk for adverse neonatal outcomes, particularly in cases with early onset proteinuria.

Majority of women with chronic hypertension during pregnancy may be in stage 1 and may only require lifestyle modifications, and careful evaluation and monitoring of blood pressures is all that may be required in most patients, particularly in the context of a physiological drop in blood pressure during the first half of pregnancy. Some physicians advocate no antihypertensive medication during pregnancy. This stems from a meta-analysis of 45 randomized controlled studies of treatment with several classes of antihypertensive drugs in stages 1 and 2 hypertension during pregnancy. This meta-analysis showed a direct linear relationship between treatment-induced fall in mean arterial pressure and the proportion of small-for-gestational-age infants. This relationship was independent of type of hypertension, type of antihypertensive agent, and duration of therapy.

However, for pregnant women with target organ damage or those who required multiple antihypertensive agents for control, antihypertensive medication should be continued as needed to control blood pressure (BP). In all cases, treatment should be re-instituted once BP reaches 150–160 mmHg systolic or 100–110 mmHg diastolic. Aggressive treatment of severe chronic hypertension in the first trimester is critical, since foetal loss rates of 50% and significant maternal mortality have been reported in these patients. Most of the poor outcomes are related to superimposed pre-eclampsia. Further, women with chronic hypertension are also at higher risk for adverse neonatal outcomes if proteinuria is present early in pregnancy.

22.5.4 **Management of pre-eclampsia**

Delivery of the baby is the definitive treatment. However, the decision to deliver would need to take into account both maternal and foetal well-being and would depend on foetal gestational age, foetal status, and severity of the maternal condition at assessment. Some indications for delivery include severe overt clinical symptoms in the mother, grossly abnormal lab tests, and foetal ill-health.

Severe pre-eclampsia requires immediate control and regular, frequent monitoring of blood pressure with high-dependency care. Anaesthetic services and, on occasions, critical care services should be involved in management at an early stage. Eclamptic seizures are associated with an unprecedented number of deaths and hence eclampsia is a serious complication that should be avoided.

22.5.5 **Pharmacologic treatment**

Antihypertensive treatment essentially prevents potential cerebrovascular and cardiovascular complications, the most common cause of maternal morbidity and mortality, and do not prevent or alter the natural course of the disease in women with mild pre-eclampsia.

Many drugs are available for the control of high blood pressure in pregnancy. A familiarity with the maternal and foetal side effects as well as their mode of action is imperative to make the right choice.

The commonly used drugs in the treatment of hypertension in pregnancy are labetalol, methyldopa, nifedipine, clonidine, diuretics, and hydralazine. Labetalol is the drug of choice for the management of hypertension in pregnancy. Magnesium sulfate is used in the management of pre-eclamptic patients to prevent eclamptic seizures. Sodium nitroprusside is the drug of choice in hypertensive crises. Nitroglycerin is a mixed arterio-venous dilator and the drug of choice in pre-eclampsia associated with pulmonary oedema and control of hypertension associated with tracheal manipulation, although it is contraindicated in hypertensive encephalopathy due to its effects on cerebral perfusion and intracranial pressure. Diuretics and calcium-channel blockers are probably safe, but there are limited data and they are not recommended as first-line agents.

Angiotensin-converting enzyme inhibitors are contraindicated in pregnancy due to high rates of foetal abnormalities and foetal death. Beta blockers are another group of drugs that are relatively contraindicated due to the higher incidence of small-for-date babies when the mothers were given these drugs. However, in case of compelling indications such as coronary artery disease, aortic dissections, and so on, beta blockers could be used where the benefits outweigh the risks.

22.6 **Hypertensive emergencies**

Hypertensive encephalopathy, acute left ventricular failure, acute aortic dissection, or increased circulating catecholamines (phaeochromocytoma, clonidine withdrawal) are acute emergencies that require urgent blood pressure lowering because of their potentially life-threatening consequences, particularly in women with underlying heart disease, chronic renal disease, multiple-drug therapy to control hypertension, superimposed pre-eclampsia in the second trimester, and abruptio placentae with disseminated intravascular coagulation (DIC).

A detailed discussion of their management is beyond the scope of this book and further reading is recommended.

22.7 **Conclusions**

Hypertension in pregnancy is an important medical condition with profound effects on the health of the mother and the foetus. Management of hypertension in pregnancy requires a multidisciplinary approach towards a safe and uneventful pregnancy and delivery.

Key references

Alexander JM, Wilson KL (2013). Hypertensive emergencies in pregnancy, *Obstetric and Gynecology clinics of North America;* 40: 89–101.

American College of Obstetricians and Gynecologists (1996). Hypertension in pregnancy. ACOG Technical Bulletin No. 219. Washington, DC: The College; 1–8.

Cantwell R, Clutton-Brock T, Cooper G, et al. (2011). Saving Mothers' Lives: Reviewing maternal deaths to make motherhood safer: 2006–2008. The Eighth Report of the Confidential Enquiries into Maternal Deaths in the United Kingdom. *British Journal of Obstetrics and Gynaecology;* 118 Suppl 1:1–203.

Coppage KH, Sibai BM (2005). Treatment of hypertensive complications in pregnancy. *Current Pharmaceutical Design;* 11: 749–57.

Karthikeyan VJ, Lip GY (2007). Hypertension in pregnancy: pathophysiology and management strategies. *Current Pharmaceutical Design;* 13: 2567–79.

Lindheimer MD (1993). Hypertension in pregnancy. *Hypertension;* 22: 127–37.

Report of the National High Blood Pressure Education Program Working group (2000). Report on high blood pressure in pregnancy. *American Journal of Obstetrics Gynecology;* 183: S1–S22.

Sibai BM (2005). Diagnosis, prevention, and management of eclampsia. *Obstetrics Gynecology;* 105(2): 402–10.

Chapter 23

Malignant hypertension

VJ Karthikeyan

Key points

- Malignant hypertension is associated with very high blood pressures and ischaemic organ damage.
- With the widespread use of antihypertensive agents its incidence is reducing but it is still associated with significant morbidity and mortality.
- Commonest presentation is headache and visual disturbances.
- Management should include continuous cardiac monitoring and frequent assessment of neurological status and urine output.
- Oral agents are as effective as intravenous agents in controlling blood pressure in this setting.

23.1 Introduction

Malignant hypertension is a syndrome of elevated blood pressure, vascular injury, and ischaemic organ damage (retina, kidney, heart or brain). The vascular injury is characterized by fibrinoid necrosis and proliferative endarteritis. It is a hypertensive emergency associated with ischaemic retinal changes consistent with grades III or IV hypertensive retinopathy (Figure 23.1).

The incidence of malignant hypertension is 1–2% per 100 000 per year, with a significant morbidity and mortality, particularly related to long-term cardiac and renal complications. One-year survival rate is 76%. It occurs in a relatively young age group and is more frequent in males, with Afro-Caribbean patients particularly at risk.

In the pre-antihypertensive treatment era, the incidence of malignant hypertension was 7% and has now dropped to 1–2% of the hypertensive population. Although its frequency is very low, the absolute number of new cases has not changed much over the past 40 years. The survival rate five years after diagnosis of malignant hypertension has improved significantly (it was close to zero 50 years ago), possibly as a result of earlier diagnosis, lower BP targets, and availability of new classes of antihypertensive agents. Although malignant hypertension can develop in patients with essential hypertension as well as those with secondary hypertension, the risk is greater in the latter group. (Some of the causes of malignant hypertension are listed in Box 23.1.) Further, it can develop at lower diastolic pressures and early in the course of the disease, suggesting that the rate of rise is more significant than absolute pressure levels.

23.2 Pathophysiology of malignant hypertension

As mentioned earlier, there are significant vascular changes seen in malignant hypertension. The characteristic vascular lesions fall into two categories. The first lesion is fibrinoid necrosis affecting the afferent arterioles and comprises transmural necrosis of the smooth muscle cells

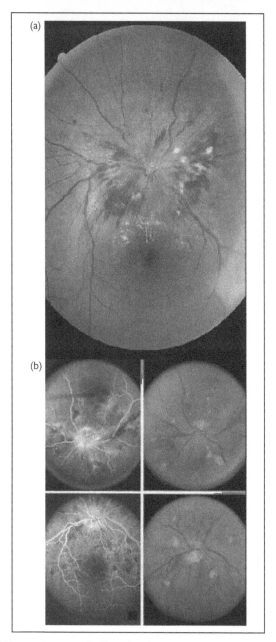

Figure 23.1 (a) Hypertensive retinopathy (flame-shaped haemorrhages, soft exudates, and blurring of the disc); (b) malignant hypertension: papilloedema (swelling of the optic disc with blurred margins).

Box 23.1 Causes of malignant hypertension

Primary
- Essential hypertension

Secondary
- Renal diseases
  - Renal parenchymal disease
  - Glomerulonephritis
  - Pyelonephritis
  - Analgesic/radiation nephropathy
  - Renal artery stenosis
  - Renal cholesterol emboli
- Endocrine causes
  - Phaeochromocytoma
  - Hyperaldosteronism
- Others
  - Scleroderma

of the arteriole combined with deposition of fibrin and platelets, with intramural haemorrhage. The endothelial cells in these vessels appear to remain viable. Fibrinoid necrosis heals by fibrous replacement of the arterial wall, with a consequent loss of haemodynamic control. The second lesion is proliferative endarteritis affecting the medium-sized to small-resistance arteries; in the kidney, these are the interlobular arteries. This lesion is characterized by a concentric 'onion skin' proliferation of smooth muscle cells and myofibroblasts. There is narrowing of the arterial lumen with consequent severe tissue ischaemia. Factors that are suggested to contribute to the vascular injury in malignant hypertension include direct pressor injury, vasculotoxic substances, volume depletion, localized intravascular coagulation, and kinins. Further, red blood cells are damaged as they flow through vessels obstructed by fibrin deposition, resulting in microangiopathic haemolytic anaemia, causing deterioration in renal function.

A loss in homeostasis (cerebral vasoconstriction maintaining cerebral perfusion in response to increases in blood pressure) occurs at high blood pressures, resulting in arteriolar dilatation, hyperperfusion, and cerebral oedema, and the clinical manifestations of hypertensive encephalopathy. Elevated peripheral plasma renin activity and increased aldosterone production are also known to occur and cause vascular damage.

23.3 **Clinical features of malignant hypertension**

The most common presentations include headaches and visual disturbances, chest pain, dyspnoea, and neurologic deficits. Neurological symptoms include occipital headache, cerebral infarction or haemorrhage, visual disturbances (including transient blindness), transient paralyses, seizures, stupor or coma, or hypertensive encephalopathy (a symptom complex of severe hypertension, headache, vomiting, visual disturbance, mental status changes, seizure, and retinopathy with papilloedema). Cardiac symptoms such as angina, myocardial infarction, and pulmonary oedema may occasionally be the main presenting symptom.

Other causes of malignant hypertension include medications or drugs such as cocaine, monoamine oxidase inhibitors (MAOIs), and oral contraceptives and withdrawal of beta blockers,

Box 23.2 Clinical findings in malignant hypertension

Cardiovascular system
- Peripheral pulses (look for radio-radial and radio-femoral delay)
- Blood pressure (both arms, to rule out aortic dissection/coarctation)
- If coarctation is suspected, measure blood pressure also in the legs
- Carotid or renal bruits
- Precordium, palpate for sustained left ventricular lift; auscultate for a third or fourth heart sound or murmurs
- Volume status, with orthostatic vital signs, examination of jugular veins, assessment of liver size, and assess for peripheral oedema and pulmonary crackles

Central nervous system
- A complete neurological examination to screen for localizing signs
- Focal neurological signs to screen for cerebral haemorrhage, infarct, or the presence of a mass
- Retinal examination, to assess for flame-shaped retinal haemorrhages, soft exudates, or papilloedema

alpha stimulants (clonidine), alcohol, and steroids. Renal disease may present as oliguria (acute renal failure). Gastrointestinal symptoms include nausea and vomiting.

The importance of a thorough physical examination that includes assessment of the cardiovascular system as well as the nervous system cannot be over-emphasized.

The common signs to look for are listed in Box 23.2.

23.4 **Management of malignant hypertension**

The management of malignant hypertension is a clinical challenge and begins with careful evaluation and appropriate investigations. A multidisciplinary approach, with advice from

Box 23.3 Complications of malignant hypertension

Cerebral damage, related to
- Coma
- Hypertensive encephalopathy
- Intracerebral haemorrhage
- Seizures
- Cerebral arterial vasoconstriction/dilatation
- Stroke
- Cerebral oedema

Myocardial damage, including
- Angina
- Myocardial infarction
- Left ventricular dysfunction
- Renal failure
- Recurrent episodes of malignant hypertension
- Permanent blindness

specialists in hypertension, renal physicians, cardiologists, and endocrinologists as appropriate is invaluable in the management of patients presenting with an acute hypertensive crisis.

Most of the organ systems, including the brain, eyes, blood vessels, heart, and kidneys are at risk of serious damage due to the extreme rise in blood pressure (Box 23.3). The blood vessels of the kidney are particularly susceptible and renal failure may develop, which may be permanent. Prompt treatment may help reduce risk of complications and permanent end organ damage.

23.4.1 **Investigations**

Initial laboratory tests should include a full blood profile (full blood count, electrolytes, renal function tests, glucose, coagulation studies) and urine analysis. Tests such as cardiac enzymes, thyroid function tests, urinary catecholamines, and vanillylmandelic acid aid in further workup towards the underlying aetiology.

Elevations in urea and creatinine, raised sodium and phosphate levels, high or low potassium levels (particularly in hyperaldosteronism, as a result of renal potassium wasting), and acidosis are some of the common findings. Proteinuria, microscopic haematuria, and red blood cell and hyaline casts in urine are typical of malignant hypertension.

Important imaging studies help in further assessing and ascertaining the cause of the malignant hypertension (for instance, a chest radiograph to assess for cardiac enlargement, pulmonary oedema, or involvement of other thoracic structures, such as rib notching with aortic coarctation or a widened mediastinum with aortic dissection; renal ultrasound scan to assess for structural abnormalities, renal angiography to assess for renal artery stenosis, computed tomography of the head to assess for intra-cranial haemorrhage or infarction or space-occupying lesions).

A 12-lead electrocardiogram is useful in assessing for cardiac ischaemia or infarct, presence of left ventricular hypertrophy, and evidence of electrolyte disturbances and effects of drug overdose.

23.4.2 **Treatment**

Patients are admitted and treated in hospital in an intensive care setting with continuous cardiac monitoring and frequent assessment of blood pressure levels, neurological status, and urine output. Alterations in the auto regulation of blood pressure occur, with aggressive attempts at lowering blood pressure resulting in organ hypoperfusion. Hence, current treatment is founded on agents that can be administered by intravenous infusion and titrated, and so can act promptly but gradually in order to avoid excessive hypotension and further ischaemic organ damage.

Initial aims directed at reducing the mean arterial pressure by approximately 25% over the first 24–48 hours (or a diastolic blood pressure of 100–110 mmHg, whichever is lower), with an intra-arterial line for continuous monitoring of blood pressure and titration of drug therapy are advised. Depletion of sodium and intravascular volume may be severe, and volume expansion with isotonic sodium chloride solution is worth considering.

Pharmacological measures

No trials exist comparing the efficacy of various agents in the treatment of malignant hypertension, in view of its low incidence. Drugs are chosen based on their rapidity of action, ease of use, and special situations (such as hypertension in pregnancy).

It must be emphasized that although malignant hypertension requires urgent treatment, it is not an indication for parenteral therapy. Oral antihypertensive treatment with a long-acting calcium-channel blocker (e.g. amlodipine or modified-release nifedipine) or a diuretic (e.g. bendroflumethiazide) may be commenced. Over the next two or three days blood pressure should be further reduced using a calcium-channel blocker, diuretic, ACE inhibitor, beta blocker, or vasodilator, alone or in combination. On the rare occasion when parenteral therapy is required, the most commonly used intravenous (IV) drug is sodium nitroprusside. Labetalol is another common drug used, providing easy transition from IV to oral (PO) dosing. Hydralazine is reserved for use in pregnant patients, while phentolamine is the drug of choice for a phaeochromocytoma crisis. Clevidipine is a new third-generation dihydropyridine calcium-channel blocker with unique pharmacodynamic and pharmacokinetic properties, that has also been shown to be useful in hypertensive emergencies.

When diuretics are insufficient to correct volume retention, ultrafiltration and temporary dialysis may be beneficial.

23.5 **Further management**

Patients are safely discharged following adequate control of blood pressure, evaluation for secondary causes of hypertension as appropriate, and supportive advice towards optimal blood pressure control and preventing further episodes of malignant hypertension.

Appropriate follow-up for close monitoring of blood pressure and titration of treatment by the patient's general practitioner or nurse specialist as well as hospital specialist review is mandatory. Patients are encouraged to self-monitor their blood pressures with validated blood pressure monitors at home as it eliminates any potential white-coat effect.

With current treatment, the incidence of serious complications is declining. Death is usually due to cardiovascular causes, although renal failure is an important factor too.

Key references

Elliot WJ (2004). Clinical features and management of selected hypertensive emergencies. *Journal of Clinical Hypertension* (Greenwich); 6: 587–92.

Lip GY, Beevers M, Beevers G (1994). The failure of malignant hypertension to decline: a survey of 24 years' experience in a multiracial population in England. *Journal of Hypertension*; 12: 1297–305.

Mancia G, Fagard R, Narkiewicz K, et al. (2013) ESH/ESC guidelines for the management of arterial hypertension: the Task Force for the Management of Arterial Hypertension of the European Society of Hypertension (ESH) and of the European Society of Cardiology (ESC). *European Heart Journal*; 34: 2159–219.

Marik PE, Rivera R (2011); Hypertensive emergencies: An update. *Current Opinion in Critical Care*; 17:569–80

Nadar S, Beevers DG, Lip GY (2005). Echocardiographic changes in patients with malignant phase hypertension: the West Birmingham Malignant Hypertension Register. *Journal of Human Hypertension*; 19: 69–75.

Sarafidis PA, Georgianos P, Malindretos P, (2012) Pharmacological management of hypertensive emergencies and urgencies: focus on newer agents. *Expert opinion on Investigational Drugs*; 18:1089–106

van den Born BJ, Koopmans RP, Groeneveld JO, et al. (2006). Ethnic disparities in the incidence, presentation and complications of malignant hypertension. *Journal of Hypertension*; 24: 2299–304.

Zampaglione B, Pascale C, Marchisio M, et al. (1996). Hypertensive urgencies and emergencies. Prevalence and clinical presentation. *Hypertension*; 27: 144–47.

Chapter 24

Treatment of the elderly patient

Mohammad Khan and Pravin Jha

> **Key points**
>
> - Hypertension, especially isolated systolic hypertension, is common in the elderly.
> - Detection is important but care must be paid to detail to avoid over-diagnosis.
> - Ambulatory blood pressure monitoring (ABPM) is recommended to confirm the diagnosis of hypertension.
> - Hypertension is a major risk factor for fatal and non-fatal stroke, major coronary events, chronic heart failure, retinopathy, and renal disease.
> - Secondary hypertension is uncommon in the elderly but treatment can unmask renovascular disease.
> - Treatment is worthwhile as even a modest decline in the blood pressure translates into major risk reduction.
> - Non-pharmacological needs should be encouraged for everyone.
> - Management can be challenging in view of the incidence of side effects, institution of polypharmacy, and increased prevalence of orthostatic hypotension.

163

24.1 Introduction

Blood pressure readings are continuous variable in the population and follow a Gaussian distribution. It is therefore not possible to define a 'normal blood pressure' but instead arbitrarily assign values above which there is increased likelihood of cardiovascular risk, and offer treatment targeted to those who have values below these in order to reduce risk.

Hypertension is common in older people and it is estimated that more than 70% of the UK population above the age of 60 would be considered hypertensive using the current British and American guidelines—greater than 140/90 mmHg. Even with a more conservative definition of 160/95 mmHg, it is estimated that more than 50% of this age group would be labelled hypertensive, the majority of these patients having isolated systolic hypertension.

24.2 Background/pathophysiology

Atherosclerosis and calcification of the peripheral arteries lead to reduced arterial compliance and a rise in the systolic blood pressure (SBP). The diastolic blood pressure (DBP) tends to fall after the age of 80 and this leads to a widened pulse pressure and isolated systolic hypertension, which are considered to be independent risk factor. Diastolic hypertension accounts for less than 10% of all patients with hypertension after age 70. Pulse pressure increases with age and has emerged as a potent risk factor for coronary artery disease events in older patients. Some studies have shown pulse pressure is a stronger risk factor than SBP, DBP or mean pressure in older adults. The ageing autonomic nervous system becomes dysfunctional and this causes problems with the response to change in posture. There is an immediate fall in systolic pressure on standing up and delayed recovery either when the posture is maintained or when supine position is assumed. This tends to limit the use of various antihypertensive drugs in this age group due to severe symptomatic postural hypotension.

24.3 Detection of hypertension

High blood pressure is generally considered to be asymptomatic. Headaches are attributed to the condition but clinical studies have not proved this. It is often asymptomatic and thus, has been referred to as a 'silent killer'. Blood pressure fluctuates with day-to-day activities and with various other natural life events and in the elderly, and these fluctuations are thought to be much greater than in the younger individuals.

Pseudo hypertension refers to a falsely increased SBP. Its occurrence in elderly varies widely ranging between 1.7% and 70%. Due to this extreme variation its actual prevalence is not clear. White-coat hypertension is also more common in elderly. Most guidelines therefore recommend ambulatory blood pressure monitoring (ABPM) to confirm the diagnosis of hypertension. If a person is unable to tolerate ABPM, the suitable alternative is home blood pressure monitoring (HBPM). While using ABPM for monitoring BP it is important to ensure that at least two measurements per hour are taken during the person's usual waking hours. A minimum of 14 measurements are needed and average calculations are taken. If HBPM is used for diagnosis of hypertension it is important to ensure that blood pressure is measured while person is seated, two consecutive measurements are taken at least 1 minute apart for each blood pressure recording. Blood pressure should be recorded twice daily for a minimum of four days. Ideally two blood pressure recordings are taken, one in the morning and one in the evening for seven days.

24.4 Benefits of treating hypertension in the elderly

The higher systolic or diastolic blood pressure in older persons, the greater the morbidity and mortality. The benefits of treating hypertension including isolated systolic hypertension up to the age of 80 years is clearly demonstrated. Studies such as the Systolic Hypertension in the elderly Programme (SHEP) study, the Systolic Hypertension Study in China (SYST-CHINA), and the Systolic Hypertension Study in Europe (SYST-EUR) demonstrated the reducing blood pressure in older adults with isolated systolic hypertension prevents stroke (relative reduction (RR) 30–38%), and renal failure. It is also a recognized risk factor for all types of cognitive impairment in late life and treatment retard the progression of disease. The relative risk reduction remains the same at all ages but as the absolute risk of complication is higher among older patients, the number needed to treat is lower in the elderly individual, that is, the benefit is more in the elderly group.

In the past, the benefit of treating high blood pressure in individuals above the age of 80 was not clear. An old meta-analysis of intervention trails that included patients aged over 80 years concluded that there was no overall benefit to mortality with active treatment, although there was a significant reduction in both fatal and non-fatal stroke and cardiovascular events, and this had guided treatment for many years. However, recently, the Hypertension in the Very Elderly Trial (HYVET) investigated this topic and has enrolled nearly 4000 patients above the age of 80 from 11 countries. The aim of the trial was to study the risks and benefits of treating these patients with diuretic-based regime (indapamide SR) versus placebo, with the addition of angiotensin-converting enzyme (ACE) inhibitor perindopril if required. This study has some important pre-specified sub-studies including those evaluating cognitive functions and arterial compliance. The primary results of the HYVET showed that active treatment resulted in: 30% reduction in the rate of fatal or non-fatal stroke (95% CI −1 to 51, $p = 0.06$), a 39 % reduction the rate of death from stroke (95% CI 1–62, $p = 0.05$), a reduction in all-cause death (95% CI 4–35, $p = 0.02$), a 23% reduction in cardiovascular death (95% CI −1 to 40, $p = 0.06$), and a 64% reduction in rate of heart failure (95% CI 42–78, $p < 0.01$). Thus antihypertensive therapy in elderly ($\geq$ 80 years) appears beneficial. The HYVET results provide clear evidence that BP lowering by drugs is associated with definitive CV benefits in patients equal to or greater than 80 years of age.

24.5 Assessment of the elderly hypertensive patient

Malignant hypertension is rare in the elderly, but presence of bilateral haemorrhages and cotton wool spots would be indicative of the diagnosis. The prognosis is poor; less than 1% survived one year without adequate treatment but 80% survive if effectively treated. If readings are greater than 180 mmHg systolic and 110 mmHg diastolic, urgent hospital admission is needed for investigation and treatment. As autoregulation of cerebral blood flow may be impaired in these patients, it is important to avoid sudden reduction in the blood pressure.

The prevalence of secondary hypertension is low in the elderly, as most causes would be expected to have been detected and dealt with earlier. However, the prevalence of renovascular diseases is higher than in the younger population and may be as much as 5% in the elderly population. Clinical clues include abdominal bruit, peripheral vascular disease, worsening renal function after the institution of ACE inhibitors or angiotensin receptor blockers (ARBs). Other conditions such as primary aldosterpnism, phaoechromocytoma, or Cushing's syndrome may occasionally be diagnosed and are potentially treatable causes of hypertension.

24.6 Management of the elderly hypertensive patient

Clinical and epidemiological studies such as the Framingham Heart Study suggest that in an elderly patient, the SBP provides more appropriate classification and risk stratification than the DBP. Pulse pressure is only marginally stronger than the systolic blood pressure for risk stratification in this age group.

NICE recommends the target clinic blood pressure below 140/90 mmHg in people aged less than 80 years, and below 150/90 mmHg in people aged 80 years and above. The European Society of Hypertension (ESH) and the European Society of Cardiology (ESC) guidelines recommend octogenarians with initial SBP greater than 160 mmHg should be treated to reduce SBP to between 150 and 140 mmHg provided they are in good physical and mental conditions. Fit elderly under the age of 80 years should be treated in the same way as the younger hypertensive patients are treated; that is, consider antihypertensive treatment if SBP is more than 140 mmHg with target SPB less than 140 mmHg if treatment is well tolerated. Frailty is common in the elderly and ESH and ESC guidelines leave the decision to the treating physician regarding starting antihypertensive therapy in the group. If the hypertensive patient is an octogenarian it is recommended to continue with the same treatment if it is well tolerated. ESC and ESH also recommends all hypertensive agents can be used to treat the elderly, but diuretics and calcium antagonists are preferred in isolated systolic hypertension. Although treatment in elderly must be individualized, the therapy can be initiated with two antihypertensive drugs if BP is more than 20/10 mmHg above the goal.

It must be remembered that even if the target is not achieved but blood pressure is lowered by 5–6 mmHg, it is worthwhile as this can achieve substantial cardiovascular risk reduction. Similarly, although there is no conclusive clinical trial data to suggest that treatment of stage 1 hypertension in the elderly is associated with cardiovascular risk reduction, the Joint National Committee on Prevention, Detection, Evaluation and Treatment of High Blood Pressure (JNC-7) recommends that treatment in this group should not be withheld on the basis of age alone. Whilst it is important to treat hypertension as part of a package addressing overall cardiovascular risk factors, there is merit in trying to achieve a simple target level for both patient and primary care physician. It is gratifying to reach the target levels and if not, attention should be focused on reviewing the reasons for not achieving the required results. There is the dilemma of how low we should go and in general, the evidence is as low as possible without side effects as there does not seem to be any indication of a J-shaped curve at which it was postulated that lowering blood pressure beyond a certain level is harmful.

24.6.1 **Non-pharmacological measures/lifestyle interventions**

Lifestyle modifications, such as reduced salt intake to less than 5 g day, increased physical activity by taking regular exercise, increased consumption of vegetables, fruits, and low-fat dairy products, smoking cessation, and controlling body weight, are as important in the elderly as they are in the rest of the population, and care must be given to educate this patient group. It is understood that due to general health and comorbidities, not all elderly hypertensive patients may be able to follow the lifestyle charges strictly, but an attempt must be made to educate them.

Salt reduction is especially important as per the Trial of Non-pharmacologic Interventions in the Elderly (TONE), reducing sodium to 2 g day reduced blood pressure by 3/2 mmHg over 30 months. This drop, however, was not associated with a reduction in cardiovascular events. Nearly half of those on low-salt diet were able to discontinue their antihypertensive medications. There was a further drop in blood pressure when weight loss was combined with salt reduction.

24.6.2 **Pharmacological measures**

Drug treatment is important in the overall management in addition to the non-pharmacological methods mentioned earlier, to try and achieve the targets recommended. The recommendations for the use of antihypertensive agents are similar to the general population. In the elderly population, the side effects of medication may be particularly significant increases morbidity at the expense of an elusive longevity is not appreciated both by the doctor and the patient. It is very important to bear this in mind rather than slavishly chase targets. A concordance between doctor and patient is more likely to aid compliance in the long run. The aim of titrating should be to 'start low and go slow'. It is very likely that the elderly would be on numerous medications and drug interactions should be actively monitored for. . However, it is equally important for them to be on medication deemed essential after careful deliberation. Treatment of comorbid illnesses dictates choice of therapeutic agent. One drug alone is less likely to achieve the target levels and most people would be on at least two medications. The use of combination tablets would be useful, as they would reduce the number of tablets to be taken. Lastly, the adage of adding life to years rather than years to life should be followed. The cornerstone of ethical medical practice is to first do no harm. The different treatment groups are discussed in the respective chapters.

24.7 **Specific problems in the elderly**

Tolerability is the main problem in treating elderly hypertensive patients as they are more prone to side effects. It is important to ask specifically about side effects during each clinical

Box 24.1 Possible reasons for inadequate response to treatment

- Low dose of medication
- Ineffective treatment
- Poor adherence to therapeutic regime
- Lifestyle issues—obesity, smoking, excessive alcohol intake, and insulin resistance
- Failure to use large enough cuff on the arm
- Drugs used concomitantly that raise blood pressure—for example, NSAIDs, steroids
- Volume overload—for example, high sodium intake, renal impairment
- Undetected secondary cause—for example, renal, endocrine

encounter and not dismiss such concerns. This aids in proactively identifying the problem and rectifying it in a timely manner and hence improve compliance.

Elderly hypertensive patients can be divided into two groups; one group is those who have grown old with their hypertension and are comfortable with their drugs and second are those who have hypertension detected when they are old. This second group may prove difficult to manage as they may resent the intrusion of lifestyle modification and drugs in their everyday life. However, much can be achieved with perseverance and patience. The role of the practice nurse is invaluable in this aspect of management. Both groups will require careful monitoring. It would be desirable to encourage the concept of the expert patient who might be prepared to give practical advice to the newly diagnosed hypertensive group. It helps to give ownership of the problem to the patients who would be better motivated in managing their life-long condition.

Compliance is often a major issue in this patient population. This must be carefully considered in those patients with difficulty in controlling blood pressure. Compliance may be hampered by the large number of tablets that are prescribed or it may be due to cognitive and/or physical limitations. Box 24.1 lists some of the common causes of failure of treatment in this group.

Postural hypotension is more common in the elderly and can present with falls or syncope. It is recommended that blood pressure be measured in the lying and standing positions especially if the patient complains of light-headedness. The approach is to minimize the dose and use graduated pressure stockings to try and prevent peripheral pooling but it can be a difficult problem to manage.

Finally, diabetes and hyperlipidaemia must be treated in older persons with hypertension as they increase risk of cardiovascular events.

24.8 Conclusions

Chronological age alone should not prevent careful management of hypertension but must be balanced against the risk in frail, house-bound individuals whose treatment is best made on the basis of carefully considered clinical judgements. However, it is in this age group that blood pressure reduction have the most benefit.

Key references

Beckett NS, Peters R, Fletcher AE, et al. (2008). Treatment of hypertension in patients 80 years of age or older. New England Journal of Medicine; 358 (18): 1887–98.

Forette F, Seux ML, Starssen JA, et al. (1998). Prevention of dementia in randomized double-blind placebo-controlled systolic hypertension in Europe (Syst-Eur) trial. Lancet; 352: 1347–51.

Gueyffier F, Bulpitt C, Boissel JP, et al. (1999), Antihypertensive drugs in very old people: a subgroup Meta-analysis of randomized controlled trials. *Lancet*; 353: 793–96.

O'Brien E, Petrie JC, Littler WA, et al. (1997). *Blood pressure measurement. Recommendation for the British Hypertension Society*. London: BMJ Publishing.

Rockwood K, Freter S (2001). Office management of elderly hypertensive patients. *Canadian Family Physician*; 47: 2520–5.

Thijs L, Fagard R, Lijneen P, et al. (1992). A meta-analysis of outcome trials in elderly hypertensive. *Journal of Hypertension*; 10: 1103–9.

NICE (2011). Hypertension—Clinical Management of Primary Hypertension in adults. August 2011 NICE Guideline.

ACCF/AHA (2011). Expert Consensus Document on Hypertension in the Elderly: A Report of the American College of Cardiology Foundation Task Force on Clinical Expert Consensus Documents. *Circulation*; 2011; 123:2434–506.

The Task Force for the management of arterial hypertension of the European Society of Hypertension (ESH) and of the European Society of Cardiology (ESC) (2013). 2013 ESH/ESC Guidelines for the management of arterial hypertension. *European Heart Journal*; 34, 2159–219.

Chapter 25

Resistant hypertension

Sunil Nadar

Key points

- Up to 40% of the hypertensive population may have resistant hypertension.
- Resistant hypertension should only be considered in those with poor control of blood pressure despite three rational antihypertensive agents, including a diuretic at maximal dose.
- Poor adherence, failure to modify lifestyle, inadequate treatment, white-coat hypertension, and secondary hypertension are all common aetiologies.
- Consider prescription of additional diuretic therapy, vasodilators, alpha blockers, and centrally acting agents.
- Referral to a specialist hypertension clinic should be considered for further investigation and/or management.

25.1 Definition

Although various definitions exist, most authorities consider resistant hypertension as failure to achieve adequate control of blood pressure despite adherence to treatment with at least three antihypertensive drugs including a diuretic at maximal dose. The diagnosis of resistant hypertension should not be reserved for those patients who are established on antihypertensive treatment but could also be used in those only recently diagnosed with hypertension. Resistant hypertension is sometimes termed 'refractory' or 'difficult-to-treat' hypertension. It is important to note that uncontrolled hypertension is not synonymous with resistant hypertension as there are many reasons why an individual patient's blood pressure may not be controlled.

25.2 Prevalence

There are large discrepancies in data from clinical trials and epidemiological surveys on the prevalence of resistant hypertension. In specialist clinics and hypertension trials, failure to achieve adequate blood pressure control despite appropriate triple-drug therapy is reported to be as great as 40% of the hypertensive population. It is thought that the prevalence of resistant hypertension is rising, but this may relate to improved access to healthcare and greater awareness of the importance of good blood pressure control amongst both physicians and patients. Resistant hypertension is more common in those over the age of 60 years and amongst those from economically deprived and ethnic backgrounds.

25.3 Aetiology

In many instances, apparently resistant hypertension is a result of poor compliance, suboptimal therapy, secondary hypertension, or white-coat hypertension. It is important therefore that each of these aetiologies be considered by appropriate history taking, physical examination, and investigation. The finding of resistant hypertension should prompt referral to a specialist hypertension service.

25.4 **Key investigations**

The diagnosis of resistant hypertension relies upon accurate assessment of blood pressure. This should be measured after the patient has been seated quietly for five minutes. The patient should be asked whether he has smoked a cigarette within the last 30 minutes as smoking causes a transient rise in blood pressure. Similarly the patient should not have consumed caffeine, although the effect of this stimulant on blood pressure is much less dramatic. The patient's arm should be supported at heart level and an appropriately sized cuff applied. The clinician should ensure that the sphygmomanometer used has been properly calibrated and is in good working order with no leaks in the rubber tubing.

Increasingly, automated devices have replaced mercury sphygmomanometers. These devices have important and recognizable benefits over their mercury-containing counterparts: avoidance of the hazards of mercury; robustness; ease of use and greater reproducibility by the unskilled operator. Nonetheless, it is important to remember that the relative simplicity of these devices does not negate the importance for good blood pressure measurement technique. One must also consider that not all devices are certified for conditions such as atrial fibrillation or pregnancy.

The use of home blood pressure monitoring or ambulatory blood pressure monitors may aid the diagnosis of white-coat hypertension and these investigations should be considered in patients with resistant hypertension—particularly when there is a gradual fall in blood pressure on serial measurements taken in the clinic. Most patients with white-coat hypertension also have raised blood pressure at baseline and it important, therefore, if this diagnosis is made that antihypertensive medications are not discontinued.

Other investigations should also be considered to ensure that secondary causes of hypertension have not been overlooked (Table 25.1). Such investigations are not necessary in all hypertensive patients, particularly when there is a strong family history of essential hypertension, but due consideration should be paid to each diagnosis, as many are treatable.

25.5 **Management**

There are limited data assessing the optimal strategy for management of resistant hypertension. Consequently, most strategies are based on observational data from case series managed within specialist hypertension clinics. The recommendations discussed here are therefore to be considered guidance only and the choice of regimen should be tailored as much as possible to the individual patient using clinical experience. In all cases, adherence to drug therapy, lifestyle modification, and the causes of secondary hypertension should be considered prior to embarking on treatment with additional pharmacological agents.

25.5.1 **Lifestyle modification**

Patients should be encouraged wherever possible to comply with lifestyle modifications. This includes restriction of salt intake (the current recommended daily allowance within the United Kingdom is 6 g/day), which offers a modest reduction in blood pressure of up to 8 mmHg. Similar reductions may be seen when alcohol intake is decreased and with regular physical activity.

Table 25.1 Causes of secondary hypertension

Clinical scenario	Disorder	Investigations
Snoring, obesity, daytime somnolence	Obstructive sleep apnoea	Sleep studies
Hypernatraemia, hypokalaemia	Primary aldosteronism	Ratio of plasma aldosterone to plasma renin activity Adrenal vein sampling CT scan of adrenal glands
Renal insufficiency, atherosclerotic cardiovascular disease, oedema, proteinuria	Renal parenchymal disease	Creatinine clearance, 24-hour urinary protein collection, renal ultrasonography
Decline in renal function on introduction of ACE inhibitor or ARB, loss of previously good blood pressure control, widespread vascular disease, abdominal bruit	Renal artery disease	Magnetic resonance angiography, renal arteriography
Weight gain, fatigue, proximal muscle weakness, amenorrhea, moon facies, dorsal hump, striae, obesity, hypokalemia, osteoporosis	Cushing's disease	Dexamethasone suppression test
Palpitations, headache, diaphoresis	Phaeochromocytoma	Raised urinary cathecholamine excretion, CT or MRI imaging
Fatigue, weight loss, hair loss, diastolic hypertension, muscle weakness	Hypothyroidism	Thyroid function tests
Weight loss, palpitations, tremor, tachycardia, systolic hypertension, exophthalmos	Hyperthyroidism	Thyroid function tests
Renal stones, osteoporosis, lethargy, muscle weakness	Hyperparathyroidism	Serum calcium, parathyroid hormone
Headaches, visual disturbance, enlargement of hands, feet, and tongue	Acromegaly	Growth hormone
Aortic coarctation	Brachial or femoral pulse delay, systolic murmur	Chest X-ray, echocardiography, MRI or CT aorta

ACE = angiotensin-converting enzyme; ARB = angiotensin receptor blocker; MRA = magnetic resonance angiography; MRI = magnetic resonance imaging; CT = computed tomography; VMA = vanillymandelic acid.

25.5.2 **Compliance**

One major contributor to poor blood pressure control is poor compliance with drug therapy. Poor compliance is often difficult to judge as the vast majority of patients claim to take all their medications regularly. However, subtle physiological signs may be present such as tachycardia despite prescription of beta blockers or a rate-limiting calcium-channel blocker. Similarly, missed clinic appointments or apparent ignorance of prescribed drugs are also suggestive. Adverse drug effects may also contribute to poor adherence to prescribed therapy and this needs evaluation.

Compliance may be improved by involvement of specialist nurse practitioners who are able to spend more time with patients reviewing side effects and reinforcing the importance of good blood pressure control. The use of multicompartment compliance aids prepared by the patient's pharmacy is also helpful in serving as a reminder to take medications on time. The use of combination drugs (e.g. a thiazide diuretic combined with an angiotensin-converting enzyme inhibitor) may also improve compliance and with some drugs reduces overall cost.

25.5.3 **Pharmacological agents**

Diuretics

Patients with resistant hypertension frequently remain volume overloaded despite the use of either a thiazide or loop diuretic. One of the most important strategies therefore is to opti-mize volume status with additional or increased diuretic therapy and over 60% of patients will respond to this approach. In most patients, the diuretic of choice is a thiazide, although in patients with concomitant heart failure or lower glomerular filtration, loop diuretics are pre-ferred. Short-acting loop diuretics (e.g. furosemide, bumetanide) should be used in split doses to maximize effect, and minimize reac-tive sodium retention mediated by the renin–angioten-sin–aldosterone system. Naturally, use of high-dose or combination diuretic therapy requires close observation of renal function and serum electrolytes.

Aldosterone antagonists

Primary aldosteronism is increasingly appreciated as an important secondary cause of resist-ant hypertension. Moreover, patients with resistant hypertension often have excess circulating aldosterone, despite low plasma renin activity and low sodium intake. The use of aldosterone antagonists (e.g. spironolactone 25–50 mg) in such cases has been shown to have some suc-cess with sometimes impressive reductions in blood pressure. Moreover, co-prescription of spironolactone can help ameliorate the hypokalaemia often observed with thiazide and loop diuretic therapy and it acts in synergy with drugs that modulate the renin–angiotensin cascade. Naturally, serum electrolytes must be monitored closely for signs of biochemical dehydration or hyperkalaemia when treatment must be discontinued immediately.

Alpha- and beta-adrenergic receptor blockade

Whilst no longer recommended as first-line antihypertensive agents, due to only modest blood pressure-lowering effects and potential for provoking new onset of type 2 diabetes mellitus, beta blockers remain an important component of treatment in resistant hypertension. In par-ticular, these drugs should be considered complementary to other treatments such as direct vasodilators and alpha blockers, whilst use in hypertensive patients with ischaemic heart dis-ease or arrhythmias is considered routine.

Similarly alpha-adrenergic blockers also prove useful in some patients with resistant hyper-tension by promoting peripheral vascular smooth muscle relaxation and consequent vasodilata-tion. Where possible, long-acting variants should be used to minimize reflex tachycardia due to unopposed beta activity (unless co-prescription of a beta blocker). The use of alpha blockers can also be problematic in women, however, due to deterioration in bladder control resulting in incontinence.

In phaeochromocytoma, alpha blockade remains an important treatment strategy prior to definitive treatment with surgical removal of the adenoma. Once adequate alpha blockade has been established, beta blockers are introduced with caution to control the tachycardia.

Direct vasodilators

The direct vasodilators hydralazine and minoxidil are used in some patients with resistant hyper-tension and can give impressive results. However, these drugs are often poorly tolerated by the patient due to flushing, sodium and water retention, and reflex tachycardia. Consequently, rate-limiting drugs (e.g. beta blocker) and diuretics should be used in combination. In addition, minoxidil can result in the idiosyncratic onset of pericardial effusion, whilst hydralazine can provoke idiopathic systemic lupus erythematosis. Hence the use of these drugs is generally reserved under specialist guidance.

Centrally acting agents

Several centrally acting antihypertensive drugs are available. Amongst the most commonly used are methyldopa, moxonidine, and clonidine. However, side effects with each of these drugs are common, with only a modest impact on blood pressure, unless high doses are used.

Direct renin blockers

Only one drug, aliskiren, is currently licensed in this new class of agents that directly inhibit the activity of renin upstream. In clinical trials, aliskiren has been tested alone and in combination with other agents, namely, hydrochlorthiazide and valsartan. In each study, aliskiren did offer further reductions in blood pressure, with a favourable side-effect profile and therefore prescription in patients with resistant hypertension would seem reasonable. However, clinical experience remains limited.

Specific interventions

Surgical intervention should be considered in those with primary aldosteronism, phaeochromocytoma, and Cushing's disease. However, this may depend on the presence of an identifiable tumour following imaging studies and consequently specialist review is required. Surgical removal of the tumour may not lead to complete resolution of hypertension and often patients still require one or more antihypertensive drugs.

In renal artery stenosis, angioplasty and stenting have been cited as potential treatments to improve blood pressure and renal function. However, the results from case series are less encouraging with (slightly) improved blood pressure control seen in only around 50% of patients. Improvements in renal function and rate of deterioration are even less modest. However, ongoing trials are assessing the potential efficacy of this treatment in a more structured manner.

In obstructive sleep apnoea, patients may receive benefit from continuous positive airways pressure (CPAP) delivery through a tight-fitting nasal mask. The pressure delivered provides a pneumatic stent, thereby maintaining patency of the upper airways during sleep when the natural tone of the airway musculature reduces predisposing to collapse. CPAP has been shown to reduce snoring and reduce the occurrence of apnoeic episodes. This translates into improved sleep, reduced daytime somnolence, and better blood pressure control. Unfortunately, use of CPAP is often precluded by cost, whilst compliance rates are low because of poor patient tolerance.

25.6 **Renal artery denervation**

Catheter-based renal artery sympathetic denervation is a novel technique that appears to be effective in lowering blood pressure in patients with resistant hypertension. In the Symplicity HT1 trial, three -year follow-up data were presented in 88 patients who were followed up for 36 months. There was a drop of around 32 mmHg systolic and 14 mmHg diastolic at 36 months. Drops of 10 mmHg or more in systolic blood pressure were seen in 69% of patients at 1 month, 81% at 6 months, 85% at 12 months, 83% at 24 months, and 93% at 36 months. This offers an interesting avenue to explore in patients with proven resistant hypertension. This is further explained in more detail in chapter 18.

25.7 **Summary**

Resistant hypertension is common, and given the major contribution of blood pressure to cardiovascular ill health, requires prompt recognition and treatment. In particular, it is important to recognize that resistant blood pressure, although usually the result of poor adherence, may be due to secondary hypertension and should prompt relevant investigation in appropriate cases.

Key references

Amar J (2007). Patients with resistant hypertension. *Journal of Hypertension Supplement*; 25(Suppl 1): S3–6.

Calhoun DA., Jones D, Texter S, *et al.* (2008) Resistant Hypertension: Diagnosis, Evaluation, and Treatment: A Scientific Statement from the American Heart Association Professional Education Committee of the Council for High Blood Pressure Research. *Circulation*; 117:e510–e526

de la Sierra A, Segura J, Banegas JR, *et al.* (2011). Clinical features of 8295 patients with resistant hypertension classified on the basis of ambulatory blood pressure monitoring. *Hypertension*; 57(5):898.

Hirsch S (2007). A different approach to resistant hypertension. *Cleveland Clinic Journal of Medicine*; 74(6): 449–56.

Krum H, Schlaich MP, Böhm M, *et al.*. (2013). Percutaneous renal denervation in patients with treatment-resistant hypertension: final 3-year report of the Symplicity HTN-1 study. *Lancet*; Nov 6. pii:S0140-6736(13)62192–3.

Moser M, Setaro JF (2006). Clinical practice. Resistant or difficult-to-control hypertension. *New England Journal of Medicine*; 355: 385–92.

O'Rorke JE, Richardson WS (2001). Evidence based management of hypertension: what to do when blood pressure is difficult to control. *British Medical Journal*; 322: 1229–32.

Chapter 26

Hypertension in diabetic patients

Vasudevan A Raghavan and Sunil Nadar

> ## Key points
>
> - Hypertension occurs frequently in diabetics and is often associated with macro and microvascular complications.
> - Volume expansion, hyperinsulinaemia, the renin–angiotensin system, and increased arterial stiffness play a role in the pathogenesis of the complications of the hypertensive diabetic patient.
> - Management of these patients encompasses reduction of cardiovascular risk and the reduction of target organ damage (TOD). The target blood pressure values are lower than for non-diabetic hypertensive patients.
> - Angiotensin-converting enzyme (ACE) inhibitors or angiotensin-receptor blockers (ARBs) should be used as first-line therapy, either as monotherapy or usually in combination with other agents to help reduce blood pressure and prevent renal complications.

26.1 Introduction

A worldwide epidemic of diabetes mellitus (DM) is emerging. It has been estimated that by the year 2025, there will be 300 million people in the world with DM. Of these individuals, 97% will have type 2 diabetes mellitus (T2DM), which is strongly associated with visceral obesity and insulin resistance. These patients will experience multiple microvascular (retinopathy, nephropathy, and neuropathy) and macrovascular complications, although the latter accounts for more than 70% of DM associated mortality. Hypertension often coexists with DM and is a significant contributor to cardiovascular disease (CVD) in those with DM. For this reason, early recognition and energetic management of hypertension in individuals is warranted in every individual who carries the dual diagnoses of DM and hypertension.

26.2 Epidemiology of diabetes and hypertension

Hypertension tends to occur more frequently in those with DM, and those with hypertension are two-and-a-half times more likely to develop DM within five years of diagnosis. Hypertension prevalence rates in those with T2DM may approach 80% in many European countries, and a vast majority of such patients have a blood pressure (BP) greater than or equal to 140/90 mmHg. In those with T1DM, hypertension is highly prevalent as well, with the incidence rising from 5% at 10 years to 33% at 20 years, and can be as high as 70% at 40 years. The absence of normal nocturnal 'dipping' of BP in DM patients is linked to other CVD surrogates such as left ventricular hypertrophy (LVH) and microalbuminuria. The coexistence of hypertension and DM predisposes to all forms of CVD (coronary artery disease (CAD), peripheral arterial disease (PAD), and stroke), progression of renal disease,

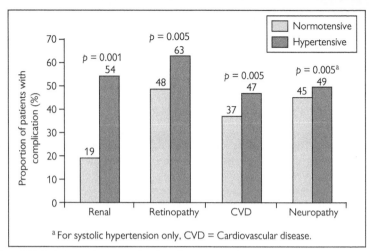

Figure 26.1 Diabetic complications attributed mainly to coexistent hypertension
Adapted from: Mehler PS, *et al.* (1997). *American Journal of Hypertension*, 10: 152–61.

and diabetic retinopathy. Numerous clinical trials have shown that blood pressure and CVD events/mortality are highly correlated in those with DM, as are hypertension and development/progression of nephropathy, retinopathy, and blindness. The presence of hypertension adversely influences overall mortality in DM by four- to fivefold by exacerbating cardiomyopathy and renal failure and is a major determinant of heart failure that is very common in those with DM. From data drawn from death certificates, hypertension has been implicated in 44% of deaths coded to DM, and DM is involved in 10% of deaths coded to hypertension. It has been estimated that 35–75% of diabetic complications can be attributed mainly to coexistent hypertension (Figure 26.1).

There is also a close relation between hypertension and renal disease in those with T1DM (Box 26.1). The BP typically begins to rise within the normal range about three years after the onset of microalbuminuria. Ultimately, the incidence of hypertension is approximately 15–25% of all patients with microalbuminuria and 75–85% in those with overt diabetic nephropathy. In the UK Prospective Diabetes Study (UKPDS), which enrolled those with T2DM only, hypertension was present in about 40% of patients at diagnosis, increasing to 80–90% when diabetic nephropathy (urinary albumin excretion > 300 mg/day) developed. In the 'Hypertension in Diabetes' study of 3500 newly diagnosed diabetic patients, 39% were already hypertensive at the time of recruitment. In approximately 50% of these patients, the elevation in BP occurred before the onset of microalbuminuria. Hypertension was strongly associated with obesity, and increased CVD-related complications. The risk of hypertension was highest in blacks, who were also at much greater risk for diabetic nephropathy end-stage renal disease (ESRD). Box 26.1 outlines important differences in T1DM and T2DM with respect to prevalence of albuminuria, hypertension, and renal failure.

26.3 **Pathophysiology**

Although several mechanisms (Table 26.1) apart from diabetic nephropathy have been proposed for the pathogenesis of hypertension in diabetes, the following merit a brief discussion.

Box 26.1 Differences between type 1 and type 2 diabetes in the evolution of proteinuria and renal disease

Type 1
- Diagnosis of hypertension does not precede onset of persistent proteinuria
- Hypertension present at onset of diabetic nephropathy in at least half of patients
- Hypertension almost always present at time of end-stage renal failure
- Microalbuminuria always presages progressive renal dysfunction
- Persistent proteinuria never detected at onset of clinical diabetes

Type 2
- Diagnosis of hypertension precedes onset of persistent proteinuria in about 20–30% of cases
- Hypertension present at onset of diabetic nephropathy in more than half of patients
- Microalbuminuria does not always presage progressive renal dysfunction
- Persistent proteinuria detected in about 10% of cases at onset of clinical diabetes

Common to both type 1 and type 2
- Hypertension almost always present at time of end stage renal failure
- Microalbuminuria presages diabetic nephropathy in about 80% of cases
- Microalbuminuria predicts cardiovascular mortality
- Hypertension exacerbates diabetic nephropathy
- Hypertension treatment slows progress of diabetic nephropathy

Table 26.1 Typical profile of blood pressure regularity	
Factor	Typical findings in hypertensive diadetics
Total exchangeable sodium	Typically increased
Plasma renin activity	Low normal to low
Plasma norepinephrine	Usually normal in nonazotemic nonketotic patients
Plasma aldosterone	Low to normal low
Baroreceptor sensitivity	Typically decreased
Vascular compliance	Typically decreased
Peripheral vascular resistance	Typically increased
Vascular pressor responses	Typically increased
Evidence of renal dysfunction	Typically present in type I patients
Central adiposity	Often increased in type II patients
Insulin resistance	Typically increased in type II patients
Abnormal cation transport mechanisms	Often present in both type I and II diabetic states

Adapted from Epstein, M and Sowers, JR (1992). Diabetes mellitus and hypertension. *Hypertension*, **19**(5): 403–18.

26.3.1 **Hyperinsulinaemia**

Insulin resistance (IR) is an important determinant in the development and progression of diabetic microvascular and macrovascular complications. Hyperinsulinaemia, either due to IR in T2DM or to insulin administration, may increase systemic BP. Insulin's hypertensive response, although not noted in all studies, may be due to concurrent weight gain and in part, due to its intrinsic effect on vasculature. Hyperinsulinaemia may be a link to explain the association between obesity and hypertension both in non-diabetic patients and those with T2DM, since insulin can increase sympathetic activity and promote renal sodium retention.

26.3.2 Volume expansion

Sodium retention and volume expansion may be induced by both insulin and the hyperglycemia-induced increase in filtered glucose load (hyperactive filtration). The excess filtered glucose is reabsorbed (as long as there is only moderate hyperglycemia) in the proximal tubule via a sodium–glucose cotransporter, resulting in a parallel rise in sodium re-absorption. The hypertensive effects of salt loading can be reversed by salt restriction. Active weight loss, by decreasing hyperinsulinaemia, will also amplify benefits by reducing insulin-mediated salt loading.

26.3.3 Increased arterial stiffness

Patients with DM have increased vascular stiffness, thought to be due to increased protein glycation and eventually atheroma formation. The reduction in arterial distensibility, which is seen with both impaired glucose tolerance and overt diabetes, can contribute to the rise in systolic pressure and is associated with mortality risk.

26.3.4 Renin–angiotensin system (RAS) abnormalities

Plasma renin activity (PRA) levels in DM tend to be variable. In part, these differences are due to patient-related factors, age and diet being two of them. PRA is usually low in patients with diabetic nephropathy and retinopathy. PRA suppression could be due to volume expansion and increased intracellular availability of calcium, an ion known to modulate vascular reactivity. Neural factors play a role in renin release, as evidenced by the fact that DM patients with autonomic neuropathy tend to have lower PRA. Overall, in the absence of microvascular complications, most diabetic patients have normal PRA.

Serum levels of angiotensin-converting enzyme (ACE) may be elevated in those with DM, even in those with low PRA, perhaps reflecting microvascular damage/endothelial dysfunction. Angiotensin II, because of its effects on the mesangial movement of macromolecules, may influence progression of diabetic nephropathy, independent of hypertension. Increased levels of inactive renin have been reported in literature, suggesting an inability to normally activate renin and may contribute to changes in PRA in diabetic patients.

26.3.5 Hyperglycaemia

Chronic hyperglycaemia contributes to hypertension in diabetic individuals. Sodium retention and an increase in exchangeable body sodium, as alluded to earlier, are important factors. In experimental animals rendered diabetic by streptozotocin, this mechanism is efficient, rapidly operative, and insulin independent. Thus, sodium retention may occur even in those with mild-to-moderate hyperglycaemia. Chronic hyperglycaemia is endothelial cell-toxic and results in increased vascular rigidity, decreased endothelial-mediated vascular relaxation, increased vasoconstriction, promotion of vascular smooth muscle cell hyperplasia, and vascular remodelling (Figure 26.2).

High glucose levels mimicking the diabetic hyperglycaemic state have also been shown to enhance expression of fibronectin and collagen IV. In the kidney, these compounds cause thickening of glomerular basement membrane and mesangial expansion. Hyperglycaemia also accelerates formation of non-enzymatic advanced glycosylation products, which accumulate in vessel wall proteins in proportion with time-integrated blood glucose concentration. An

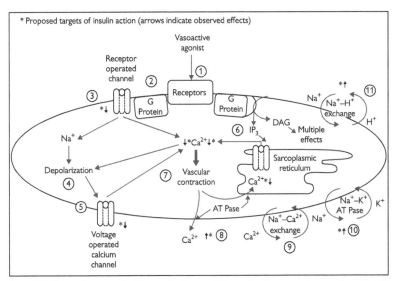

Figure 26.2 Schematic diagram depicting mechanisms regulating contraction in vascular smooth muscle cells and proposed targets of insulin action.

From Sowers JR; Epstein M; Froehlich ED. Diabetes, hypertension, and cardiovascular disease: an update. *Hypertension* 2001 Apr; 37(4):1053–9. Schematic diagram depicting mechanisms regulating contraction in vascular smooth muscle cells and proposed targets of insulin action. Pivotal steps in regulation of contraction are indicated by circled numbers.

increased level of advanced glycosylation end products correlates greatly with the incidence of new vascular complications. A membrane-associated macrophage receptor that specifically recognizes proteins to which advanced glycosylated end products are bound has recently been described. The receptor–ligand interaction induces the synthesis and secretion of tumour necrosis factors, interleukin-1, and other cytokines, which in turn stimulate other cells to increase protein synthesis and to proliferate. Interleukin-1 causes vascular smooth muscle cells, mesangial cells, and endothelial cells to proliferate and increases glomerular Type IV collagen synthesis. Interleukin-1 and other cytokines induce the expression of the proto-oncogenes c-myc and c-fos, and the growth-promoting effects of tumour necrosis factors and insulin seem to be synergistic. Thus, prolonged hyperglycaemia could lead to expansion of extracellular matrix and vascular smooth muscle proliferation and vascular remodelling. Eventually, enhanced vasoconstriction and accelerated atherogenesis and microvascular compromise ensue. A minor but intriguing mechanism may be hyperglycaemia induced irreversible non-enzymatic glycosylation of apolipoproteins conferring increased particle atherogenicity. Receptor-mediated uptake of these modified lipoproteins may be impaired, resulting in prolonged plasma retention, thereby enhancing phagocytosis and 'foam cell' formation.

26.4 **Complication of hypertension in patients with diabetes mellitus**

Clinical trial data show a close correlation between BP and CVD morbidity and mortality, development and progression of nephropathy, and progression of retinopathy and development of blindness. In the UKPDS study, every 10 mmHg decrease in mean systolic pressure was associated with reduced risk by 12% for any diabetic complication, 15% for diabetes-related deaths, 11% for myocardial infarction, 13% for macrovascular complications, and a no-risk threshold was found for any endpoint studies. The Appropriate Blood Pressure Control in Diabetes (ABCD) clinical trial tested the primary hypothesis that intensive (as opposed to moderate) BP control would prevent or slow the progression of diabetic nephropathy, neuropathy, retinopathy, and cardiovascular events. In the ABCD trial, at enrolment, nephropathy, retinopathy, cardiovascular disease, and neuropathy were significantly more prevalent in those with DM and hypertension (diastolic blood pressure > 90 mmHg) than in those with DM and diastolic BP between 80–90 mmHg.

26.5 **Treatment principles**

Hypertension in the setting of DM is a multifactorial disease. Several clinical trials have shown that optimal BP control will likely need multiple agents. One estimate of the average number of antihypertensive agents needed to reach these treatment goals is around 3.4 (Figure 26.3); the use of two or more complementary agents may improve response rates by acting on diverse pathophysiologic pathways that collude to produce hypertension in a diabetic individual. Also, combination therapy has the advantage of achieving therapeutic synergy while minimizing dose-dependant adverse effects of the individual drugs. In the Hypertension Optimal Treatment (HOT) Study, 74% of study participants needed to take two or more antihypertensive agents to lower their diastolic BP to 80 mmHg or less, and the cardioprotective effect of low-dose combination therapy exceeded that of higher-dose monotherapy. Likewise, in the United Kingdom Prospective Diabetes Study, 29% of patients in the tight BP control group required treatment with three or more medications to achieve a BP of 144/82 mmHg and reduce DM-related complications and death.

An equally important principle is to aggressively address all CVD risk factors in those with DM. In the Multiple Risk Factor Interventional Trial (MRFIT), absolute risk of CVD death was much higher for diabetic than non-diabetic men of every age stratum, ethnic background, and risk-factor level (Figure 26.4).

26.5.1 **Non-pharmacologic therapy**

According to the American Heart Association and the American Diabetes Association 2007 guidelines, non-pharmacologic methods may be particularly appropriate for all diabetic patients with a systolic blood pressure of 130–139 mmHg or a diastolic pressure of 80–89 mmHg.

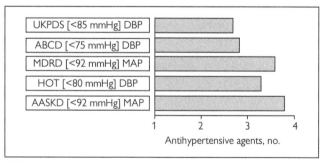

Figure 26.3 Cardiovascular and renal trials in which patients received two or more antihypertensive agents for intensive target blood pressure control

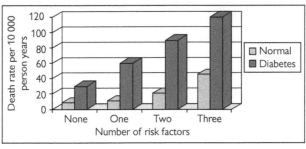

Figure 26.4 Death rate per 10 000 people

Adapted from: Stamler J, Vaccaro O, Neaton JD, Wentworth D. Diabetes, other risk factors, and 12-yr cardiovascular mortality for men screened in the Multiple Risk Factor Intervention Trial. Diabetes Care. 1993 Feb; **16**(2): 434–44 with permission from the American Diabetes Association, © 1993.

These measures include weight loss to achieve normal weight status, dietary sodium restriction, incorporating fresh fruits, vegetables, and low-fat dairy products in the diet, regular exercise, avoiding excess ethanol ingestion, and smoking cessation.

However, non-pharmacologic measures per se is unlikely to reduce BP in all patients. If target BP is not achieved after three months, treatment with pharmacological agents should be initiated. In addition, in anyone with BP elevations, it would be prudent to initiate on lifestyle measures and drug therapy simultaneously.

26.5.2 **Choice of drug therapy**

Studies comparing the effects of specific classes of drugs in the management of hypertension in patients with DM are summarized in Table 26.2.

Many antihypertensive agents are currently available and the initial choice would depend on the comorbidity profile of the patient, drug-tolerance issues, and the presence or absence of a 'compelling reason' as suggested by the British Hypertension Society guidelines or the use of any one class of agents. Studies of hypertension control in DM show a consistent effect: better control of BP means significantly reduced risk for CVD events and death. Also, aggressive hypertension control reduces the risk for microvascular events, including end-stage functional impairment (ESRD, blindness, etc.) in those with DM and the benefits seen are substantially greater than those seen in those with similar BP levels, but without DM.

BP targets for patients with DM should be aggressive. In the HOT study, a four-point difference in diastolic BP (85 mmHg vs 81 mmHg) resulted in a 50% decrease in risk for CVD events in patients with DM. In contrast, HOT study participants without DM received no benefit. Current evidence suggests that the diastolic BP goal in patients with T2DM should be 80 mmHg; ongoing studies may suggest an even lower diastolic target. The evidence base for setting systolic BP target goals is sparse, but a ten-point reduction in the UKPDS (154 mmHg vs. 144 mmHg) and a four-point reduction in the HOT trial (144 mmHg vs 140 mmHg) led to significant reduction in DM-related mortality and cardiovascular endpoints.

Earlier guidelines had suggested that in diabetic patients a target SBP of < 130 mmHg should be attained as it was thought that studies indicated that the lower the blood pressure achieved, the better the clinical outcomes. However, the latest guidelines by the European Society of Hypertension has suggested that no study has actually proven a benefit in diabetic patients with a blood pressure of less than 130 mmHg systolic. Therefore the current guidelines only recommend a reduction to below 140 mmHg systolic as with non-diabetics.

Table 26.2 Managing hypertension in patients with diabetes mellitus

Trial	Intervention	Relative risk		
		CVD events	Total mortality	Microvascular events
ABCD	Enalapril vs nisoldipine	0.43 (0.25–0.73)	0.77 (0.36–1.67)	Not reported
ALLHAT	Lisinopril vs chlortalidone	1.08 (1.00–1.17)	1.02 (0.91–1.13)	Not reported
	Amlodipine vs chlortalidone	1.06 (0.98–1.15)	0.96 (0.87–1.07)	Not reported
CAPPP	Captopril vs thiazide diuretic or beta blocker	0.59 (0.38–0.91)	0.54 (0.31–0.96)	Not reported
FACET	Fosinopril vs amlodipine	0.49 (0.26–0.95)	0.81 (0.22–3.02)	Not reported
IDNT (3 GROUPS)	Irbesartan vs placebo	0.91 (0.72–1.14)	0.92 (0.69–1.23)	0.80 (0.66–0.97)§
	Amlodipine vs placebo	0.88 (0.69–1.12)	0.88 (0.66–1.19)	1.04 (0.86–1.25)§
	Irbesartan vs amlodipine	1.03 (0.81–1.31)	1.04 (0.77–1.40)	0.77 (0.63–0.93)§
INSIGHT	Nifedipine GITS vs coamilozide	0.99 (0.69–1.42)	0.75 (0.52–1.09)	Not reported
LIFE	Losartan vs atenolol	0.76 (0.58–0.98)	0.06 (0.02–0.10)	#
NORDIL	Diltiazem vs beta blocker or diuretics	1.01 (0.66–1.53)	1.07 (0.63–1.84)	Not reported
STOP-2 (3 GROUPS)	Calcium-channel blocker vs diuretics or beta blockers	0.91 (0.66–1.26)	0.79 (0.54–1.14)	Not reported
	ACE inhibitor vs diuretics or beta blocker	0.85 (0.62–1.18)	0.88 (0.62–1.26)	Not reported
	ACE inhibitor vs calcium-channel blocker	0.94 (0.67–1.32)‡	1.14 (0.78–1.67)	Not reported
UKPDS	Captopril vs atenolol	1.29 (0.92–1.81)	1.14 (0.81–1.61)	1.29 (0.80–2.10)

* Values in parentheses are 95% CIs. ABCD: appropriate blood pressure control in diabetes; ACE:-angiotensin-converting enzyme; ALLHAT: Antihypertensive and Lipid-Lowering Treatment to Prevent Heart Attack Trial; CAPPP: Captopril Prevention Project; FACET: Fosinopril versus Amlodipine Cardiovascular Events Trial; GITS: gastrointestinal therapeutic system; IDNT: Irbesartan Diabetic Nephropathy Trial; INSIGHT: International Nifedipine GITS Study: Intervention as a Goal in Hypertension Treatment; LIFE: Losartan Intervention for Endpoint Reduction; NORDIL: Nordic diltiazem; STOP-2: Swedish Trial in Old Patients with Hypertension-2; UKPDS: United Kingdom Prospective Diabetes Study.

‡ The risk for myocardial infarction in the ACE inhibitor group was 0.51 (CI, 0.28–0.92) compared with the calcium-channel blocker group.

§ Composite microvascular end point—doubling of serum creatinine concentration plus development of end-stage renal disease plus all-cause mortality; individually, only

doubling of the serum creatinine concentration was statistically significantly lower with irbesartan compared with either placebo or amlodipine.

Risk for microalbuminuria was lower in the losartan group, although the risk/hazard ratio (HR) is not presented (P = 0.002). (Adapted from: Vijan S, Hayward RA.

Treatment of hypertension in type 2 diabetes mellitus: blood pressure goals, choice of agents, and setting priorities in diabetes care. Ann Intern Med. Apr 1 2003; 138(7): 593–602).

Choice of initial BP agent in patients with DM is difficult to define precisely. The weight of current evidence suggests that angiotensin II-receptor blockers (ARBs), thiazide diuretics, and ACE inhibitors (ACEI) are reasonable first-choice agents, although they are considerably more expensive than diuretics (some ACEI are now off patent). However, high doses of thiazide diuretics ought to be avoided because of lack of incremental benefit and higher incidence of metabolic complications such as worsening hyperglycaemia and dyslipidemia, hypokalaemia, hyperuricaemia, and hypercalcaemia.

Available data suggest that ARBs reduce the risk for adverse renal outcomes. In the LIFE study, ARB were superior to beta blockers in reducing CVD event rates and mortality, at least in those with electrocardiography evidence of left ventricular hypertrophy. Evidence comparing ACEI, diuretics, and beta blockers is less definitive. While the ALLHAT study found that diuretics were equivalent to ACEI for most outcomes and were superior for heart failure, the CAPPP trial found that ACEI were superior to beta blockers and diuretics. The UKPDS and STOP-2 study found that ACEI were as efficacious as beta blockers and diuretics. The HOPE study showed a hypertension-independent benefit of ACEI on mortality. However, such benefits were unapparent in ALLHAT, suggesting that factors other than BP may have played a part in the high-risk enrollees. Limited evidence suggests that ACE inhibitors may have hypertension-independent renoprotective effects in patients with DM. There are yet no long-term outcome trials comparing ARB with ACEI in those with DM and hypertension. Early data on renal outcomes and effects on intermediate endpoints such as BP control seem to be similar, although ARB may be slightly better tolerated.

Beta blockers and calcium-channel blockers have proven efficacy compared with placebo, and the evidence suggests that they are similarly efficacious. However, data (albeit less robust) suggest that diuretics, ARB, and ACEI inhibitors may be superior to beta blockers and calcium-channel blockers in those who have DM and hypertension, and as such the latter two agents ought to be second- or third-line agents of choice. Beta blockers are safe, effective, and inexpensive and at moderate doses have relatively few side effects. In the UKPDS, however, enrollees taking beta blockers gained more weight and required the addition of new glucose-lowering agents more frequently than those taking ACEI. However, the evidence base for the notion that beta blockers increase risk for hypoglycemia or hypoglycemia unawareness is sparse. Some data suggest that, in the general population, calcium-channel blockers may be more effective in reducing stroke than other agents, but this has not been definitively shown in patients with DM. The guidelines also mention that two blockers of the RAAS should be avoided in diabetics

Although this chapter has focused predominantly on T2DM, those with T1DM are at even greater risk for premature CVD. Therefore CVD risk reduction should be integral to managing the T1DM patient, principally through lifestyle modification in childhood, and then drug therapies for BP and lipids in adulthood. The ten-year Pittsburgh study which followed up people with T1DM demonstrated that BP, lipids, and concomitant peripheral vascular or renal disease are important risk factors for the prediction of CVD.

Treatment of hypertension in diabetics has been shown to reduce or delay microalbuminuria. However there are no studies that demonstrate any benefit on diabetic retinopathy or neuropathy by the treatment of hypertension.

26.6 Conclusion

A comprehensive cardiovascular risk assessment approach is necessary to lower the incidence and prevalence of cardiovascular complications in individuals with DM. The clinical trial evidence for prevention of CVD in diabetes is largely based on single-risk factor interventions. However, the Steno-2 study from Denmark has provided some evidence for the cardiovascular benefits following a multifactorial intervention programme. This trial randomized 160 adults with T2DM and microalbuminuria to a conventional or an intensive, multifactorial, goal-targeted strategy for a period of eight years. All subjects in both groups received an ACEI or ARB. In the 'targeted, intensified, multifactorial intervention group', a stepwise treatment plan was adopted for each of 4 factors; with the goals of reducing HbA1c to < 6.5% (with diet, exercise, metformin, sulfonylurea, and various insulin preparations), blood pressure to < 130/80 mmHg (with a variety of antihypertensive agents added to the ACE-I or ARB), fasting serum total cholesterol to < 175 mg/dL (with statins), and fasting serum triglycerides to < 150 mg/dL (with fibrates). All patients in the intensive group also received aspirin, regardless of whether there was a history of coronary heart disease or peripheral vascular disease. The primary endpoint was a macrovascular outcome: a composite of death from cardiovascular causes, nonfatal myocardial infarction, coronary artery bypass grafting, percutaneous transluminal coronary angioplasty, non-fatal stroke, amputation for ischemia, or vascular surgery for peripheral arterial atherosclerosis. The secondary endpoints were microvascular outcomes: the development of diabetic nephropathy (24-h urine albumin > 300 mg) or development or progression of diabetic retinopathy or neuropathy. Patients receiving intensive therapy had a significantly lower risk of cardiovascular disease (hazard ratio, 0.47; 95% confidence interval, 0.24–0.73), nephropathy (hazard ratio, 0.39; 95% confidence interval, 0.17–0.87), retinopathy (hazard ratio, 0.42; 95% confidence interval, 0.21–0.86), and autonomic neuropathy (hazard ratio, 0.37; 95% confidence interval, 0.18–0.79). The STENO-2 protocol did not confine the practitioner to any one specific algorithm, suggesting that a pragmatic 'ends justifies means' approach is plausible and

may indeed be beneficial in the high-risk T2DM patients.

Regular physician visits are mandatory for the diabetic hypertensive patient in order to screen for complications, review treatment targets, and plan effective, comprehensive, individualized care. Hypertension management has to be integrated with achieving optimal glycaemic control, and the management of other diabetic complications such as diabetic retinopathy, microalbuminuria/proteinuria, and erectile dysfunction. Most people with DM will need evidence-based polypharmacy; besides antihypertensive therapy, aspirin, metformin (T2DM) and a statin or combination lipid lowering therapy may all be required. Aggressive management of all CVD risk factors is key to minimizing morbidity and mortality in those who have diabetes and hypertension.

Key references

American Diabetes Association. Standards of medical care in diabetes—2013. *Diabetes Care;* 2013;36 (suppl 1):S11–S66.

Bakris GL (2001). A practical approach to achieving recommended blood pressure goals in diabetic patients. *Archives of Internal Medicine;* 10–24 161(22): 2661–7. Review.

Bangalore S, Parkar S, Grossman E, *et al.* (2007). A meta-analysis of 94 492 patients with hypertension treated with beta blockers to determine the risk of new-onset diabetes mellitus. *American Journal of Cardiology;* 15 100(8): 1254–62.

British Cardiac Society; British Hypertension Society; Diabetes UK; HEART UK; Primary Care Cardiovascular Society; Stroke Association (2005). Joint British Societies' guidelines on prevention of cardiovascular disease in clinical practice. *Heart;* Dec; 91(Suppl 5): v1–52.

Epstein M, Sowers JR (1992). Diabetes mellitus and hypertension. *Hypertension;* May; 19(5): 403–18.

Estacio RO, Jeffers BW, Hiatt WR, *et al.* (1998). The effect of nisoldipine as compared with enalapril on cardiovascular outcomes in patients with non-insulin-dependent diabetes and hypertension. *New England Journal of Medicine;* 5 Mar; 338(10): 645–52.

James PA, Oparil S, Carter BL, *et al.* (2014). Evidence-Based Guideline for the Management of High Blood Pressure in Adults: Report From the Panel Members Appointed to the Eighth Joint National Committee (JNC 8) *Journal of the American Medical Association;* 311(5):507–20.

Hansson L, Zanchetti A, Carruthers G, *et al.* (1998). for the Hypertension Optimal Treatment (HOT) Study Group. Effects of intensive blood-pressure lowering and low-dose aspirin in patients with hypertension: principal results of the HOT randomised trial. *Lancet*; 351: 1755–62.

Hunsicker LG, Adler S, Caggiula A (1997). Predictors of the progression of renal disease in the Modification of Diet in Renal Disease Study, *Kidney International*; 51: 1908–19.

Lindholm LH (2000). The outcome of STOP-Hypertension-2 in relation to the 1999 WHO/ISH hypertension guidelines. *Blood Pressure Supplement*; 2: 21–4.

Lindholm LH, Ibsen H, Borch-Johnsen K, *et al.* (2002). Risk of new-onset diabetes in the Losartan Intervention For Endpoint reduction in hypertension study. *Journal of Hypertension*; Sep; 20(9): 1879–86.

Mogensen CE, Hansen KW, Pedersen MM, *et al.* (1991). Renal factors influencing blood pressure threshold and choice of treatment for hypertension in IDDM. *Diabetes Care*; Nov; 14(Suppl 4): 13–26.

Reboldi G, Gentile G, Angeli F, *et al.* (2011) Effects of intensive blood pressure reduction on myocardial infarction and stroke in diabetes: a meta-analysis in patients. *Journal of Hypertension*; 29:1253–69.

The ACCORD Study Group (2010). Effects of intensive blood-pressure control in type 2 diabetes mellitus. *New England Journal of Medicine*; 362:1575–85.

The Task Force for the management of arterial hypertension of the European Society of Hypertension (ESH) and of the European Society of Cardiology (ESC) (2013). 2013 ESH/ESC Guidelines for the management of arterial hypertension. *Journal of Hypertension*; 31:1281–357.

United Kingdom Prospective Diabetes Study (UKPDS) Group (1998). Tight blood pressure control and risk of macrovascular and microvascular complications in type 2 diabetes: UKPDS 38. *British Medical Journal*; 317: 703–13.

Vijan S, Hayward RA (2003). Treatment of hypertension in type 2 diabetes mellitus: blood pressure goals, choice of agents, and setting priorities in diabetes care. *Annals of Internal Medicine*; 138(7): 593–602.

Wright JT, Jr, Bakris G, Greene T, *et al.* (2005). African American Study of Kidney Disease and Hypertension Study Group. Effect of blood pressure lowering and antihypertensive drug class on progression of hypertensive kidney disease: results from the AASK trial. *Journal of American Medical Association*; 20 Nov; 288(19): 2421–31. Erratum in: *JAMA*. 2006; 295(23): 2726.

Index

Page numbers in *italic* indicate boxes, figures and tables